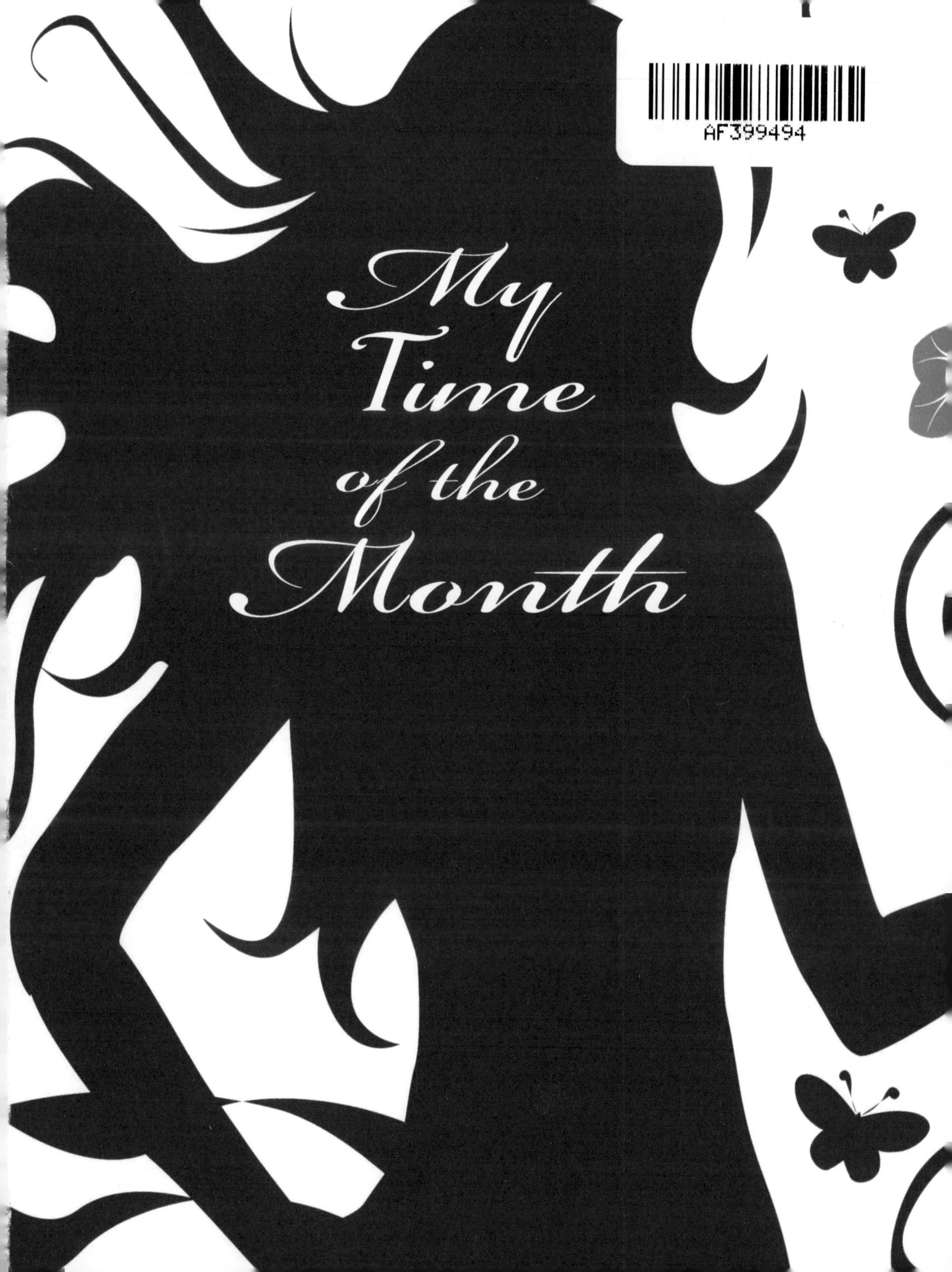
My
Time
of the
Month

Bibliografische Information der Deutschen Nationalbibliothek
Die Deutsche Nationalbibliothek verzeichnet diese Publikation in der Deutschen Nationalbibliografie; detaillierte bibliografische Daten sind im Internet über http://dnb.d-nb.de abrufbar.

My Time of the Month – Cycle Chart
Author: Dr. Caroline Oblasser

First published in German in March 2012: „Alle meine Tage – Menstruationskalender"
First English edition: March 2015, translated by Deborah Neiger (Midwife)

© 2012–2015   edition riedenburg
Address   edition riedenburg, Anton-Hochmuth-Strasse 8, A–5020 Salzburg
E-Mail   verlag@editionriedenburg.at

Internet   editionriedenburg.at
Editors   Anna Rockel-Loenhoff, Unna; Dr. Heike Wolter, Regensburg

Coverdesign, composition and layout: edition riedenburg
Girl with dog + Illustrations © Vanessa – Fotolia.com

ISBN 978-3-902943-92-7

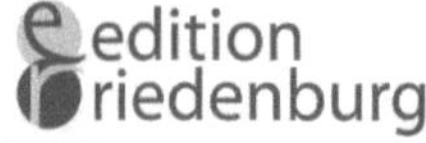

Please record the contents of this diary here,
so it is easier to locate a particular cycle:

Cycle (Dates, notes)	Page

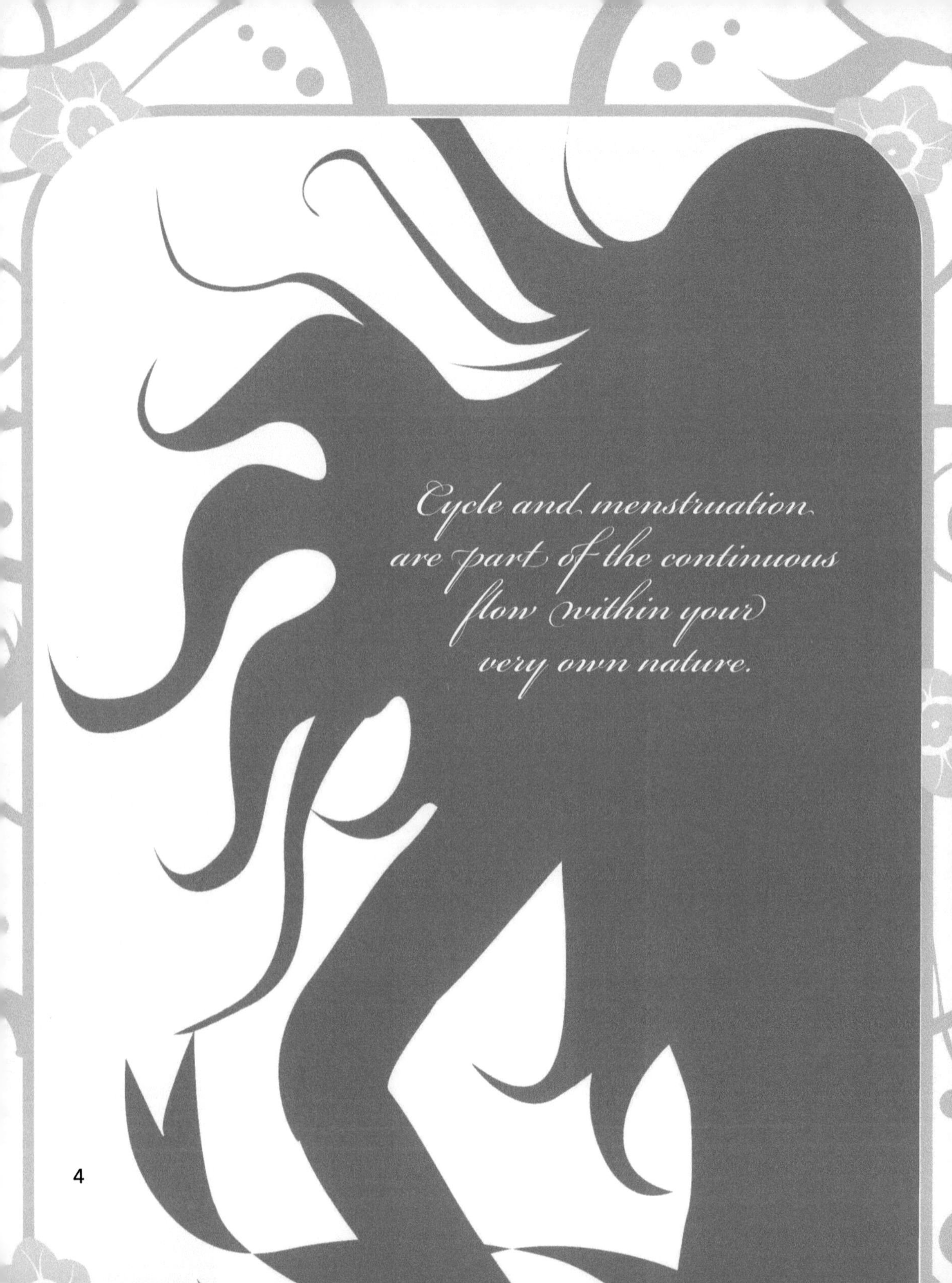
Cycle and menstruation
are part of the continuous
flow within your
very own nature.

Period timing, the wish to conceive and contraception

How do you know when your period will start? Perhaps you are one of those women who know to the minute when their period will start. Or perhaps your period regularly takes you by surprise and you are annoyed that you missed all the signs again.

Charting your cycle can help, in a very straightforward fashion, to reliably predict the start of your next period.

Take your temperature on waking before you have moved around, eaten breakfast or brushed your teeth, preferably while still lying in bed. As soon as your temperature curve takes a downturn, your period is about to start and the unfertilised egg is expelled from your body, together with the menstrual fluid.

On the following pages you can record your cycle by noting down your waking temperature, and become a pro at interpreting the signs your body is sending you.

You will find that going to bed late or alcohol consumption during the previous evening falsifies your waking temperature, making it higher. But practice makes perfect and soon no one will be able to tell you anything about your cycle you don't already know.

Conveniently, you will also be able to use your charts as a tool to avoid or achieve pregnancy.

To avoid a pregnancy, avoid sex without contraception for several days before and after ovulation. To achieve pregnancy, have sex during those very days.

The start of your fertile days is usually signalled by an increase in cervical mucus which becomes more and more stretchy and resembles eggwhite in consistency around the time of ovulation. If your egg remains unfertilised this build up of mucus is excreted together with menstrual fluid which is why you often find mucus in your menstrual blood.

Practical tip: There is plenty of charting software for different computers and mobile phones, that enable you to record waking temperature, mucus consistency and other observations. Search for 'sympto-thermal method' or 'natural family planning' for plenty of helpful results. There are lots of in depth online sources of information or books on the subject that help you narrow down your fertile period even more to either avoid or achieve a pregnancy.

Sample Cycle

Shortest cycle so far: **26** days

Longest cycle so far: **34** days

Where was temperature taken:
- Rectum ☒
- Vagina ☐
- Mouth ☐
- Ear ☐

First day of cycle: **25** . **04** . 20 **15**   Thermometer: **Digital**

Date	25.04.2015	26	27	28	29	30	1	2	3	4	5	6	7	8	9	10	11	12	13	14	15	16	17	18	19	20	21	22	23	24	25	26	27	28	29	30	31	1	2	3
Cycle-Day	1	2	3	4	5	6	7	8	9	10	11	12	13	14	15	16	17	18	19	20	21	22	23	24	25	26	27	28	29	30	31	32	33	34	35	36	37	38	39	40
Bleeding	▓	▓	▓	▓	▓																								▓											
Sex/intercourse (X)			X	X	X															X				X	X			X	X	X										
Cervical mucus (m = moist, s = sticky, e = eggwhite)						∅	∅	m	m	e	e	e	e	e	e	e	e	s	s	∅	∅																			
Ovulation (O)														O																										

Temperature chart (My waking temperature in the morning, also known as basal temperature):

| 37,5 |
| 37,4 |
| 37,3 |
| 37,2 |
| 37,1 |
| **37,0** |
| 36,9 |
| 36,8 |
| 36,7 |
| 36,6 |
| 36,5 |
| 36,4 |
| 36,3 |
| 36,2 |
| 36,1 |

Countdown numbers written on chart (around cycle-days 8–15): 8 7 6 5 4 3 2 1

Time of measuring	7	6:45	7	7	7	9	9	7	6:30	7	7:15	6:30	7	7:15	7	7	6:30	7	6:15	7	8	7	9	7	6:30	7	7:15	6	6:30	7										
Cycle-Day	1	2	3	4	5	6	7	8	9	10	11	12	13	14	15	16	17	18	19	20	21	22	23	24	25	26	27	28	29	30	31	32	33	34	35	36	37	38	39	40
Alcohol?					Wine																																			
Party, late bedtime?					Late Party																																			
Ill? Fever?																																								
Breast-feeding? (exclusive/complementary)																																								
Other notes									Ovulation pain																															

Avoiding pregnancy or wanting to achieve one? Some stats on fertility:

Earliest high temperature reading in this cycle on day: 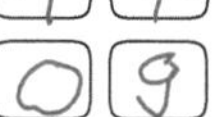

Earliest high temperature reading in all previous cycles including this one:

Deduct 8 to determine the start of your potentially fertile days = the earliest potentially fertile day so far:

Tip: Also record your ovulation day as per your own estimation and gut feeling, as well as the day determined by waking temperature, in the ovulation column. Some women are very aware of their ovaries around the time of ovulation (pulling or stabbing sensation on the right or left, just below the umbilicus). Additionally, around the time of ovulation, your cervical mucus is slippery-stretchy, almost liquid, similar to eggwhite.

You might also notice a difference in your breasts which you may want to note down on your chart.

Every cycle is different. This is why the chart on the opposite page is simply an example to illustrate filling it in. You will have to record a few cycles until you are fully familiar with your particular cycle pattern. You will notice that the temperature on day 6 and 7 of the example chart was unusually high and has therefore been put into brackets and was not counted as true 'thermal shift'. The reasons for this random rise in temperature were going to bed late and alcohol consumption the nights before. The temperature was also taken later than normal at 9am.

You will also see that a temperature shift of more than 2/10th of a degree occurred on day 17 (circled), 2 days after the estimated and felt time of ovulation (O). The cervical mucus confirms that this was the transition from fertile to infertile period: it turned from e = eggwhite consistency into s = sticky consistency on day 18.

From when on and for how long are you fertile? We can assume that a woman is infertile **after** ovulation including peak cervical mucus day, from the third evening after the true thermal shift until the start of her next period. In our example chart, this would be from the evening of cycle day 19 until cycle day 29. The first 6 days of the following cycle (cycle start: true thermal shift to lower temperatures after a period of higher ones including the start of menstruation) can also be considered infertile.

Once you are very familiar with your cycle and your cycle is very regular, your will likely be able to stretch out your infertile period **at the beginning of each cycle** for longer with careful observation of mucus, temperature and ovulation symptoms. However, **before** ovulation, there is always the theoretical potential for conception. You should most certainly consider this if you are definitely trying to avoid conception and await the more accurate infertile period in the second half of your cycle. You have to remember that sperm can survive in your body for a few days and that ovulation can be somewhat unpredictable. So you need a few days as additional 'buffer' (minus 8-rule) to avoid unwanted pregnancy. The use of condoms is of course possibly during your fertile period, but you would be relying on the contraceptive properties of the condom rather than the certainty of your own body's cycle. However, a condom can provide some, but not 100%, protection from sexually transmitted infections.

By the way: Women used to take their temperature and wonder why they ended up with an accidental pregnancy anyway. Today we know that temperature charting alone is NOT enough for safe contraception. Observing your cervical mucus is absolutely necessary to determine fertile and infertile days. With a little bit of practice you will soon be able to differentiate between different types of cervical mucus, possibly by its smell, but certainly by its consistency (sticky and tacky: not very fertile, stringy and slippery: very fertile). You can even let your partner in on the secrets of cervical mucus.

Drop in temperature = Start of period: The chart on the opposite page records a drop in temperature on day 30, which equals the start of menstruation and therefore a new cycle. The old cycle in our example had 29 days, but you will likely find that you have cycles significantly longer or shorter than this. Chart for yourself and find out what happens in your body and what course your own cycles take.

Cycle number: ☐

Shortest cycle so far: ________ days

Longest cycle so far: ________ days

Where was temperature taken:
Rectum ☐
Vagina ☐
Mouth ☐
Ear ☐

First day of cycle: _____ . _____ . 20 _____   Thermometer: ___________________

Cycle-Day	1	2	3	4	5	6	7	8	9	10	11	12	13	14	15	16	17	18	19	20	21	22	23	24	25	26	27	28	29	30	31	32	33	34	35	36	37	38	39	40
Bleeding																																								
Sex/intercourse (X)																																								
Cervical mucus m = moist s = sticky e = eggwhite																																								
Ovulation (O)																																								

My waking temperature in the morning (also known as basal temperature)

| | 37,5 |
| 37,4 |
| 37,3 |
| 37,2 |
| 37,1 |
| **37,0** |
| 36,9 |
| 36,8 |
| 36,7 |
| 36,6 |
| 36,5 |
| 36,4 |
| 36,3 |
| 36,2 |
| 36,1 |

Time of measuring

Cycle-Day	1	2	3	4	5	6	7	8	9	10	11	12	13	14	15	16	17	18	19	20	21	22	23	24	25	26	27	28	29	30	31	32	33	34	35	36	37	38	39	40
Alcohol?																																								
Party, late bedtime?																																								
Ill? Fever?																																								
Breast-feeding? (exclusive/complementary)																																								
Other notes																																								

Avoiding pregnancy or wanting to achieve one? Some stats on fertility:

Earliest high temperature reading in this cycle on day:

Earliest high temperature reading in all previous cycles including this one:

Deduct 8 to determine the start of your potentially fertile days = the earliest potentially fertile day so far:

Tip: Also record your ovulation day as per your own estimation and gut feeling, as well as the day determined by waking temperature, in the ovulation column. Some women are very aware of their ovaries around the time of ovulation (pulling or stabbing sensation on the right or left, just below the umbilicus). Additionally, around the time of ovulation, your cervical mucus is slippery-stretchy, almost liquid, similar to eggwhite.

Sanitary protection used in this cycle:

Pain levels and/or pain medication used in this cycle:

My experiences with freebleeding in this cycle:

Wishing to avoid/achieve pregnancy in this cycle:

Anything else of importance in this cycle:

Cycle number: [ ]

Shortest cycle so far: _________ days

Longest cycle so far: _________ days

Where was temperature taken:
Rectum ☐
Vagina ☐
Mouth ☐
Ear ☐

First day of cycle: _____ . _____ . 20 _____   Thermometer: _________________

Cycle-Day	1	2	3	4	5	6	7	8	9	10	11	12	13	14	15	16	17	18	19	20	21	22	23	24	25	26	27	28	29	30	31	32	33	34	35	36	37	38	39	40
Bleeding																																								
Sex/intercourse (X)																																								
Cervical mucus m = moist s = sticky e = eggwhite																																								
Ovulation (O)																																								

My waking temperature in the morning (also known as basal temperature)

37,5
37,4
37,3
37,2
37,1
37,0
36,9
36,8
36,7
36,6
36,5
36,4
36,3
36,2
36,1

Time of measuring

Cycle-Day	1	2	3	4	5	6	7	8	9	10	11	12	13	14	15	16	17	18	19	20	21	22	23	24	25	26	27	28	29	30	31	32	33	34	35	36	37	38	39	40
Alcohol?																																								
Party, late bedtime?																																								
Ill? Fever?																																								
Breast-feeding? (exclusive/ complementary)																																								
Other notes																																								

Avoiding pregnancy or wanting to achieve one? Some stats on fertility:

Earliest high temperature reading in this cycle on day: ▢ ▢

Earliest high temperature reading in all previous cycles including this one: ▢ ▢

Deduct 8 to determine the start of your potentially fertile days = the earliest potentially fertile day so far: ▢ ▢

Tip: Also record your ovulation day as per your own estimation and gut feeling, as well as the day determined by waking temperature, in the ovulation column. Some women are very aware of their ovaries around the time of ovulation (pulling or stabbing sensation on the right or left, just below the umbilicus). Additionally, around the time of ovulation, your cervical mucus is slippery-stretchy, almost liquid, similar to eggwhite.

Sanitary protection used in this cycle:

Pain levels and/or pain medication used in this cycle:

My experiences with freebleeding in this cycle:

Wishing to avoid/achieve pregnancy in this cycle:

Anything else of importance in this cycle:

Cycle number: [ ]

Shortest cycle so far: ________ days

Longest cycle so far: ________ days

Where was temperature taken:
Rectum ☐
Vagina ☐
Mouth ☐
Ear ☐

First day of cycle: _____ . _____ . 20 _____   Thermometer: ___________________

Cycle-Day	1	2	3	4	5	6	7	8	9	10	11	12	13	14	15	16	17	18	19	20	21	22	23	24	25	26	27	28	29	30	31	32	33	34	35	36	37	38	39	40
Bleeding																																								
Sex/intercourse (X)																																								
Cervical mucus m = moist s = sticky e = eggwhite																																								
Ovulation (O)																																								

My waking temperature in the morning (also known as basal temperature)

37,5																																								
37,4																																								
37,3																																								
37,2																																								
37,1																																								
37,0																																								
36,9																																								
36,8																																								
36,7																																								
36,6																																								
36,5																																								
36,4																																								
36,3																																								
36,2																																								
36,1																																								

Time of measuring																																								

Cycle-Day	1	2	3	4	5	6	7	8	9	10	11	12	13	14	15	16	17	18	19	20	21	22	23	24	25	26	27	28	29	30	31	32	33	34	35	36	37	38	39	40
Alcohol?																																								
Party, late bedtime?																																								
Ill? Fever?																																								
Breast-feeding? (exclusive/complementary)																																								
Other notes																																								

Avoiding pregnancy or wanting to achieve one? Some stats on fertility:

Earliest high temperature reading in this cycle on day:

Earliest high temperature reading in all previous cycles including this one:

Deduct 8 to determine the start of your potentially fertile days = the earliest potentially fertile day so far:

Tip: Also record your ovulation day as per your own estimation and gut feeling, as well as the day determined by waking temperature, in the ovulation column. Some women are very aware of their ovaries around the time of ovulation (pulling or stabbing sensation on the right or left, just below the umbilicus). Additionally, around the time of ovulation, your cervical mucus is slippery-stretchy, almost liquid, similar to eggwhite.

Sanitary protection used in this cycle:

Pain levels and/or pain medication used in this cycle:

My experiences with freebleeding in this cycle:

Wishing to avoid/achieve pregnancy in this cycle:

Anything else of importance in this cycle:

Cycle number: [ ]

Shortest cycle so far: _______ days

Longest cycle so far: _______ days

Where was temperature taken:
Rectum ☐
Vagina ☐
Mouth ☐
Ear ☐

First day of cycle: _____ . _____ . 20 _____   Thermometer: _______________

Cycle-Day	1	2	3	4	5	6	7	8	9	10	11	12	13	14	15	16	17	18	19	20	21	22	23	24	25	26	27	28	29	30	31	32	33	34	35	36	37	38	39	40
Bleeding																																								
Sex/inter-course (X)																																								
Cervical mucus m = moist s = sticky e = eggwhite																																								
Ovulation (O)																																								

My waking temperature in the morning (also known as basal temperature)

| 37,5 |
| 37,4 |
| 37,3 |
| 37,2 |
| 37,1 |
| **37,0** |
| 36,9 |
| 36,8 |
| 36,7 |
| 36,6 |
| 36,5 |
| 36,4 |
| 36,3 |
| 36,2 |
| 36,1 |

Time of measuring

Cycle-Day	1	2	3	4	5	6	7	8	9	10	11	12	13	14	15	16	17	18	19	20	21	22	23	24	25	26	27	28	29	30	31	32	33	34	35	36	37	38	39	40
Alcohol?																																								
Party, late bedtime?																																								
Ill? Fever?																																								
Breast-feeding? (exclusive/ complementary)																																								
Other notes																																								

Avoiding pregnancy or wanting to achieve one? Some stats on fertility:

Earliest high temperature reading in this cycle on day:

Earliest high temperature reading in all previous cycles including this one:

Deduct 8 to determine the start of your potentially fertile days = the earliest potentially fertile day so far:

Tip: Also record your ovulation day as per your own estimation and gut feeling, as well as the day determined by waking temperature, in the ovulation column. Some women are very aware of their ovaries around the time of ovulation (pulling or stabbing sensation on the right or left, just below the umbilicus). Additionally, around the time of ovulation, your cervical mucus is slippery-stretchy, almost liquid, similar to eggwhite.

Sanitary protection used in this cycle:

Pain levels and/or pain medication used in this cycle:

My experiences with freebleeding in this cycle:

Wishing to avoid/achieve pregnancy in this cycle:

Anything else of importance in this cycle:

Cycle number: [ ]

Shortest cycle so far: _______ days

Longest cycle so far: _______ days

Where was temperature taken:
Rectum ☐
Vagina ☐
Mouth ☐
Ear ☐

First day of cycle: ____ . ____ . 20 ____   Thermometer: _________________

Cycle-Day	1	2	3	4	5	6	7	8	9	10	11	12	13	14	15	16	17	18	19	20	21	22	23	24	25	26	27	28	29	30	31	32	33	34	35	36	37	38	39	40
Bleeding																																								
Sex/intercourse (X)																																								
Cervical mucus m = moist s = sticky e = eggwhite																																								
Ovulation (O)																																								

My waking temperature in the morning (also known as basal temperature)

37,5
37,4
37,3
37,2
37,1
37,0
36,9
36,8
36,7
36,6
36,5
36,4
36,3
36,2
36,1

Time of measuring																																								

Cycle-Day	1	2	3	4	5	6	7	8	9	10	11	12	13	14	15	16	17	18	19	20	21	22	23	24	25	26	27	28	29	30	31	32	33	34	35	36	37	38	39	40
Alcohol?																																								
Party, late bedtime?																																								
Ill? Fever?																																								
Breastfeeding? (exclusive/complementary)																																								
Other notes																																								

Avoiding pregnancy or wanting to achieve one? Some stats on fertility:

Earliest high temperature reading in this cycle on day:

Earliest high temperature reading in all previous cycles including this one:

Deduct 8 to determine the start of your potentially fertile days = the earliest potentially fertile day so far:

Tip: Also record your ovulation day as per your own estimation and gut feeling, as well as the day determined by waking temperature, in the ovulation column. Some women are very aware of their ovaries around the time of ovulation (pulling or stabbing sensation on the right or left, just below the umbilicus). Additionally, around the time of ovulation, your cervical mucus is slippery-stretchy, almost liquid, similar to eggwhite.

Sanitary protection used in this cycle:

Pain levels and/or pain medication used in this cycle:

My experiences with freebleeding in this cycle:

Wishing to avoid/achieve pregnancy in this cycle:

Anything else of importance in this cycle:

Cycle number: [ ]

Shortest cycle so far: ________ days

Longest cycle so far: ________ days

Where was temperature taken:
Rectum ☐
Vagina ☐
Mouth ☐
Ear ☐

First day of cycle: _____ . _____ . 20 _____   Thermometer: ________________

Cycle-Day	1	2	3	4	5	6	7	8	9	10	11	12	13	14	15	16	17	18	19	20	21	22	23	24	25	26	27	28	29	30	31	32	33	34	35	36	37	38	39	40
Bleeding																																								
Sex/intercourse (X)																																								
Cervical mucus (m = moist, s = sticky, e = eggwhite)																																								
Ovulation (O)																																								

My waking temperature in the morning (also known as basal temperature)

°C	1	2	3	4	5	6	7	8	9	10	11	12	13	14	15	16	17	18	19	20	21	22	23	24	25	26	27	28	29	30	31	32	33	34	35	36	37	38	39	40
37,5																																								
37,4																																								
37,3																																								
37,2																																								
37,1																																								
37,0																																								
36,9																																								
36,8																																								
36,7																																								
36,6																																								
36,5																																								
36,4																																								
36,3																																								
36,2																																								
36,1																																								

Time of measuring																																								

Cycle-Day	1	2	3	4	5	6	7	8	9	10	11	12	13	14	15	16	17	18	19	20	21	22	23	24	25	26	27	28	29	30	31	32	33	34	35	36	37	38	39	40
Alcohol?																																								
Party, late bedtime?																																								
Ill? Fever?																																								
Breast-feeding? (exclusive/ complementary)																																								
Other notes																																								

Avoiding pregnancy or wanting to achieve one? Some stats on fertility:

Earliest high temperature reading in this cycle on day:

Earliest high temperature reading in all previous cycles including this one:

Deduct 8 to determine the start of your potentially fertile days = the earliest potentially fertile day so far:

Tip: Also record your ovulation day as per your own estimation and gut feeling, as well as the day determined by waking temperature, in the ovulation column. Some women are very aware of their ovaries around the time of ovulation (pulling or stabbing sensation on the right or left, just below the umbilicus). Additionally, around the time of ovulation, your cervical mucus is slippery-stretchy, almost liquid, similar to eggwhite.

Sanitary protection used in this cycle:

Pain levels and/or pain medication used in this cycle:

My experiences with freebleeding in this cycle:

Wishing to avoid/achieve pregnancy in this cycle:

Anything else of importance in this cycle:

Cycle number: [ ]

Shortest cycle so far: _______ days

Longest cycle so far: _______ days

Where was temperature taken:
Rectum ☐
Vagina ☐
Mouth ☐
Ear ☐

First day of cycle: _____ . _____ . 20 _____   Thermometer: __________________

Cycle-Day	1	2	3	4	5	6	7	8	9	10	11	12	13	14	15	16	17	18	19	20	21	22	23	24	25	26	27	28	29	30	31	32	33	34	35	36	37	38	39	40
Bleeding																																								
Sex/intercourse (X)																																								
Cervical mucus m = moist s = sticky e = eggwhite																																								
Ovulation (O)																																								

My waking temperature in the morning (also known as basal temperature)

37,5	
37,4	
37,3	
37,2	
37,1	
37,0	
36,9	
36,8	
36,7	
36,6	
36,5	
36,4	
36,3	
36,2	
36,1	

Time of measuring

Cycle-Day	1	2	3	4	5	6	7	8	9	10	11	12	13	14	15	16	17	18	19	20	21	22	23	24	25	26	27	28	29	30	31	32	33	34	35	36	37	38	39	40
Alcohol?																																								
Party, late bedtime?																																								
Ill? Fever?																																								
Breast-feeding? (exclusive/complementary)																																								
Other notes																																								

Avoiding pregnancy or wanting to achieve one? Some stats on fertility:

Earliest high temperature reading in this cycle on day:

Earliest high temperature reading in all previous cycles including this one:

Deduct 8 to determine the start of your potentially fertile days = the earliest potentially fertile day so far:

Tip: Also record your ovulation day as per your own estimation and gut feeling, as well as the day determined by waking temperature, in the ovulation column. Some women are very aware of their ovaries around the time of ovulation (pulling or stabbing sensation on the right or left, just below the umbilicus). Additionally, around the time of ovulation, your cervical mucus is slippery-stretchy, almost liquid, similar to eggwhite.

Sanitary protection used in this cycle:

Pain levels and/or pain medication used in this cycle:

My experiences with freebleeding in this cycle:

Wishing to avoid/achieve pregnancy in this cycle:

Anything else of importance in this cycle:

Cycle number: [ ]

Shortest cycle so far: ________ days

Longest cycle so far: ________ days

Where was temperature taken:
Rectum ☐
Vagina ☐
Mouth ☐
Ear ☐

First day of cycle: _____ . _____ . 20 _____   Thermometer: ________________

Cycle-Day	1	2	3	4	5	6	7	8	9	10	11	12	13	14	15	16	17	18	19	20	21	22	23	24	25	26	27	28	29	30	31	32	33	34	35	36	37	38	39	40
Bleeding																																								
Sex/inter-course (X)																																								
Cervical mucus m = moist s = sticky e = eggwhite																																								
Ovulation (O)																																								

My waking temperature in the morning (also known as basal temperature)

37,5	
37,4	
37,3	
37,2	
37,1	
37,0	
36,9	
36,8	
36,7	
36,6	
36,5	
36,4	
36,3	
36,2	
36,1	

Time of measuring

Cycle-Day	1	2	3	4	5	6	7	8	9	10	11	12	13	14	15	16	17	18	19	20	21	22	23	24	25	26	27	28	29	30	31	32	33	34	35	36	37	38	39	40
Alcohol?																																								
Party, late bedtime?																																								
Ill? Fever?																																								
Breast-feeding? (exclusive/complemen-tary)																																								
Other notes																																								

Avoiding pregnancy or wanting to achieve one? Some stats on fertility:

Earliest high temperature reading in this cycle on day:

Earliest high temperature reading in all previous cycles including this one:

Deduct 8 to determine the start of your potentially fertile days = the earliest potentially fertile day so far:

Tip: Also record your ovulation day as per your own estimation and gut feeling, as well as the day determined by waking temperature, in the ovulation column. Some women are very aware of their ovaries around the time of ovulation (pulling or stabbing sensation on the right or left, just below the umbilicus). Additionally, around the time of ovulation, your cervical mucus is slippery-stretchy, almost liquid, similar to eggwhite.

Sanitary protection used in this cycle:

Pain levels and/or pain medication used in this cycle:

My experiences with freebleeding in this cycle:

Wishing to avoid/achieve pregnancy in this cycle:

Anything else of importance in this cycle:

Cycle number: [ ]

Shortest cycle so far: _________ days

Longest cycle so far: _________ days

Where was temperature taken:
Rectum ☐
Vagina ☐
Mouth ☐
Ear ☐

First day of cycle: _____ . _____ . 20 _____   Thermometer: _____________________

Cycle-Day	1	2	3	4	5	6	7	8	9	10	11	12	13	14	15	16	17	18	19	20	21	22	23	24	25	26	27	28	29	30	31	32	33	34	35	36	37	38	39	40
Bleeding																																								
Sex/inter-course (X)																																								
Cervical mucus **m = moist** **s = sticky** **e = eggwhite**																																								
Ovulation (O)																																								

My waking temperature in the morning (also known as basal temperature)

| | 37,5 |
| 37,4 |
| 37,3 |
| 37,2 |
| 37,1 |
| **37,0** |
| 36,9 |
| 36,8 |
| 36,7 |
| 36,6 |
| 36,5 |
| 36,4 |
| 36,3 |
| 36,2 |
| 36,1 |

Time of measuring

Cycle-Day	1	2	3	4	5	6	7	8	9	10	11	12	13	14	15	16	17	18	19	20	21	22	23	24	25	26	27	28	29	30	31	32	33	34	35	36	37	38	39	40
Alcohol?																																								
Party, late bedtime?																																								
Ill? Fever?																																								
Breast-feeding? (exclusive/complementary)																																								
Other notes																																								

Avoiding pregnancy or wanting to achieve one? Some stats on fertility:

Earliest high temperature reading in this cycle on day:

Earliest high temperature reading in all previous cycles including this one:

Deduct 8 to determine the start of your potentially fertile days = the earliest potentially fertile day so far:

Tip: Also record your ovulation day as per your own estimation and gut feeling, as well as the day determined by waking temperature, in the ovulation column. Some women are very aware of their ovaries around the time of ovulation (pulling or stabbing sensation on the right or left, just below the umbilicus). Additionally, around the time of ovulation, your cervical mucus is slippery-stretchy, almost liquid, similar to eggwhite.

Sanitary protection used in this cycle:

Pain levels and/or pain medication used in this cycle:

My experiences with freebleeding in this cycle:

Wishing to avoid/achieve pregnancy in this cycle:

Anything else of importance in this cycle:

Cycle number: [ ]

Shortest cycle so far: ________ days

Longest cycle so far: ________ days

Where was temperature taken:
Rectum ☐
Vagina ☐
Mouth ☐
Ear ☐

First day of cycle: _____ . _____ . 20 _____   Thermometer: ___________________

Cycle-Day	1	2	3	4	5	6	7	8	9	10	11	12	13	14	15	16	17	18	19	20	21	22	23	24	25	26	27	28	29	30	31	32	33	34	35	36	37	38	39	40
Bleeding																																								
Sex/intercourse (X)																																								
Cervical mucus m = moist s = sticky e = eggwhite																																								
Ovulation (O)																																								

My waking temperature in the morning (also known as basal temperature)

	37,5	37,4	37,3	37,2	37,1	**37,0**	36,9	36,8	36,7	36,6	36,5	36,4	36,3	36,2	36,1

Time of measuring

Cycle-Day	1	2	3	4	5	6	7	8	9	10	11	12	13	14	15	16	17	18	19	20	21	22	23	24	25	26	27	28	29	30	31	32	33	34	35	36	37	38	39	40
Alcohol?																																								
Party, late bedtime?																																								
Ill? Fever?																																								
Breast-feeding? (exclusive/complementary)																																								
Other notes																																								

Avoiding pregnancy or wanting to achieve one? Some stats on fertility:

Earliest high temperature reading in this cycle on day:

Earliest high temperature reading in all previous cycles including this one:

Deduct 8 to determine the start of your potentially fertile days = the earliest potentially fertile day so far:

Tip: Also record your ovulation day as per your own estimation and gut feeling, as well as the day determined by waking temperature, in the ovulation column. Some women are very aware of their ovaries around the time of ovulation (pulling or stabbing sensation on the right or left, just below the umbilicus). Additionally, around the time of ovulation, your cervical mucus is slippery-stretchy, almost liquid, similar to eggwhite.

Sanitary protection used in this cycle:

Pain levels and/or pain medication used in this cycle:

My experiences with freebleeding in this cycle:

Wishing to avoid/achieve pregnancy in this cycle:

Anything else of importance in this cycle:

Cycle number: [ ]

Shortest cycle so far: _______ days

Longest cycle so far: _______ days

Where was temperature taken:
Rectum ☐
Vagina ☐
Mouth ☐
Ear ☐

First day of cycle: ____ . ____ . 20 ____   Thermometer: ________________

Cycle-Day	1	2	3	4	5	6	7	8	9	10	11	12	13	14	15	16	17	18	19	20	21	22	23	24	25	26	27	28	29	30	31	32	33	34	35	36	37	38	39	40
Bleeding																																								
Sex/intercourse (X)																																								
Cervical mucus m = moist s = sticky e = eggwhite																																								
Ovulation (O)																																								

My waking temperature in the morning (also known as basal temperature)

	37,5
	37,4
	37,3
	37,2
	37,1
	37,0
	36,9
	36,8
	36,7
	36,6
	36,5
	36,4
	36,3
	36,2
	36,1

Time of measuring

Cycle-Day	1	2	3	4	5	6	7	8	9	10	11	12	13	14	15	16	17	18	19	20	21	22	23	24	25	26	27	28	29	30	31	32	33	34	35	36	37	38	39	40
Alcohol?																																								
Party, late bedtime?																																								
Ill? Fever?																																								
Breast-feeding? (exclusive/complementary)																																								
Other notes																																								

Avoiding pregnancy or wanting to achieve one? Some stats on fertility:

Earliest high temperature reading in this cycle on day:

Earliest high temperature reading in all previous cycles including this one:

Deduct 8 to determine the start of your potentially fertile days = the earliest potentially fertile day so far:

Tip: Also record your ovulation day as per your own estimation and gut feeling, as well as the day determined by waking temperature, in the ovulation column. Some women are very aware of their ovaries around the time of ovulation (pulling or stabbing sensation on the right or left, just below the umbilicus). Additionally, around the time of ovulation, your cervical mucus is slippery-stretchy, almost liquid, similar to eggwhite.

Sanitary protection used in this cycle:

Pain levels and/or pain medication used in this cycle:

My experiences with freebleeding in this cycle:

Wishing to avoid/achieve pregnancy in this cycle:

Anything else of importance in this cycle:

Cycle number: [   ]

Shortest cycle so far: _________ days

Longest cycle so far: _________ days

First day of cycle: _____ . _____ . 20 _____   Thermometer: _____________________

Where was temperature taken:
Rectum ☐
Vagina ☐
Mouth ☐
Ear ☐

Cycle-Day	1	2	3	4	5	6	7	8	9	10	11	12	13	14	15	16	17	18	19	20	21	22	23	24	25	26	27	28	29	30	31	32	33	34	35	36	37	38	39	40
Bleeding																																								
Sex/intercourse (X)																																								
Cervical mucus m = moist s = sticky e = eggwhite																																								
Ovulation (O)																																								

My waking temperature in the morning (also known as basal temperature)

37,5
37,4
37,3
37,2
37,1
37,0
36,9
36,8
36,7
36,6
36,5
36,4
36,3
36,2
36,1

Time of measuring

Cycle-Day	1	2	3	4	5	6	7	8	9	10	11	12	13	14	15	16	17	18	19	20	21	22	23	24	25	26	27	28	29	30	31	32	33	34	35	36	37	38	39	40
Alcohol?																																								
Party, late bedtime?																																								
Ill? Fever?																																								
Breast-feeding? (exclusive/complementary)																																								
Other notes																																								

Avoiding pregnancy or wanting to achieve one? Some stats on fertility:

Earliest high temperature reading in this cycle on day:

Earliest high temperature reading in all previous cycles including this one:

Deduct 8 to determine the start of your potentially fertile days = the earliest potentially fertile day so far:

Tip: Also record your ovulation day as per your own estimation and gut feeling, as well as the day determined by waking temperature, in the ovulation column. Some women are very aware of their ovaries around the time of ovulation (pulling or stabbing sensation on the right or left, just below the umbilicus). Additionally, around the time of ovulation, your cervical mucus is slippery-stretchy, almost liquid, similar to eggwhite.

Sanitary protection used in this cycle:

Pain levels and/or pain medication used in this cycle:

My experiences with freebleeding in this cycle:

Wishing to avoid/achieve pregnancy in this cycle:

Anything else of importance in this cycle:

Cycle number: [ ]

Shortest cycle so far: _______ days

Longest cycle so far: _______ days

Where was temperature taken:
Rectum ☐
Vagina ☐
Mouth ☐
Ear ☐

First day of cycle: _____ . _____ . 20 ____   Thermometer: _______________

Cycle-Day	1	2	3	4	5	6	7	8	9	10	11	12	13	14	15	16	17	18	19	20	21	22	23	24	25	26	27	28	29	30	31	32	33	34	35	36	37	38	39	40
Bleeding																																								
Sex/intercourse (X)																																								
Cervical mucus m = moist s = sticky e = eggwhite																																								
Ovulation (O)																																								

My waking temperature in the morning (also known as basal temperature)

37,5
37,4
37,3
37,2
37,1
37,0
36,9
36,8
36,7
36,6
36,5
36,4
36,3
36,2
36,1

Time of measuring																																								

Cycle-Day	1	2	3	4	5	6	7	8	9	10	11	12	13	14	15	16	17	18	19	20	21	22	23	24	25	26	27	28	29	30	31	32	33	34	35	36	37	38	39	40
Alcohol?																																								
Party, late bedtime?																																								
Ill? Fever?																																								
Breast-feeding? (exclusive/ complementary)																																								
Other notes																																								

Avoiding pregnancy or wanting to achieve one? Some stats on fertility:

Earliest high temperature reading in this cycle on day:

Earliest high temperature reading in all previous cycles including this one:

Deduct 8 to determine the start of your potentially fertile days = the earliest potentially fertile day so far:

Tip: Also record your ovulation day as per your own estimation and gut feeling, as well as the day determined by waking temperature, in the ovulation column. Some women are very aware of their ovaries around the time of ovulation (pulling or stabbing sensation on the right or left, just below the umbilicus). Additionally, around the time of ovulation, your cervical mucus is slippery-stretchy, almost liquid, similar to eggwhite.

Sanitary protection used in this cycle:

Pain levels and/or pain medication used in this cycle:

My experiences with freebleeding in this cycle:

Wishing to avoid/achieve pregnancy in this cycle:

Anything else of importance in this cycle:

Cycle number: [ ]

Shortest cycle so far: _________ days

Longest cycle so far: _________ days

Where was temperature taken:
Rectum ☐
Vagina ☐
Mouth ☐
Ear ☐

First day of cycle: _____ . _____ . 20 _____   Thermometer: _______________

Cycle-Day	1	2	3	4	5	6	7	8	9	10	11	12	13	14	15	16	17	18	19	20	21	22	23	24	25	26	27	28	29	30	31	32	33	34	35	36	37	38	39	40
Bleeding																																								
Sex/intercourse (X)																																								
Cervical mucus **m = moist s = sticky e = eggwhite**																																								
Ovulation (O)																																								

My waking temperature in the morning (also known as basal temperature)

37,5
37,4
37,3
37,2
37,1
37,0
36,9
36,8
36,7
36,6
36,5
36,4
36,3
36,2
36,1

Time of measuring

Cycle-Day	1	2	3	4	5	6	7	8	9	10	11	12	13	14	15	16	17	18	19	20	21	22	23	24	25	26	27	28	29	30	31	32	33	34	35	36	37	38	39	40
Alcohol?																																								
Party, late bedtime?																																								
Ill? Fever?																																								
Breast-feeding? (exclusive/complementary)																																								
Other notes																																								

Avoiding pregnancy or wanting to achieve one? Some stats on fertility:

Earliest high temperature reading in this cycle on day:

Earliest high temperature reading in all previous cycles including this one:

Deduct 8 to determine the start of your potentially fertile days = the earliest potentially fertile day so far:

Tip: Also record your ovulation day as per your own estimation and gut feeling, as well as the day determined by waking temperature, in the ovulation column. Some women are very aware of their ovaries around the time of ovulation (pulling or stabbing sensation on the right or left, just below the umbilicus). Additionally, around the time of ovulation, your cervical mucus is slippery-stretchy, almost liquid, similar to eggwhite.

Sanitary protection used in this cycle:

Pain levels and/or pain medication used in this cycle:

My experiences with freebleeding in this cycle:

Wishing to avoid/achieve pregnancy in this cycle:

Anything else of importance in this cycle:

Cycle number: [ ]

Shortest cycle so far: ________ days

Longest cycle so far: ________ days

Where was temperature taken:
Rectum ☐
Vagina ☐
Mouth ☐
Ear ☐

First day of cycle: _____ . _____ . 20 ____   Thermometer: _________________

Cycle-Day	1	2	3	4	5	6	7	8	9	10	11	12	13	14	15	16	17	18	19	20	21	22	23	24	25	26	27	28	29	30	31	32	33	34	35	36	37	38	39	40
Bleeding																																								
Sex/intercourse (X)																																								
Cervical mucus m = moist s = sticky e = eggwhite																																								
Ovulation (O)																																								

My waking temperature in the morning (also known as basal temperature)

37,5
37,4
37,3
37,2
37,1
37,0
36,9
36,8
36,7
36,6
36,5
36,4
36,3
36,2
36,1

Time of measuring

Cycle-Day	1	2	3	4	5	6	7	8	9	10	11	12	13	14	15	16	17	18	19	20	21	22	23	24	25	26	27	28	29	30	31	32	33	34	35	36	37	38	39	40
Alcohol?																																								
Party, late bedtime?																																								
Ill? Fever?																																								
Breast-feeding? (exclusive/complementary)																																								
Other notes																																								

Avoiding pregnancy or wanting to achieve one? Some stats on fertility:

Earliest high temperature reading in this cycle on day:

Earliest high temperature reading in all previous cycles including this one:

Deduct 8 to determine the start of your potentially fertile days = the earliest potentially fertile day so far:

Tip: Also record your ovulation day as per your own estimation and gut feeling, as well as the day determined by waking temperature, in the ovulation column. Some women are very aware of their ovaries around the time of ovulation (pulling or stabbing sensation on the right or left, just below the umbilicus). Additionally, around the time of ovulation, your cervical mucus is slippery-stretchy, almost liquid, similar to eggwhite.

Sanitary protection used in this cycle:

Pain levels and/or pain medication used in this cycle:

My experiences with freebleeding in this cycle:

Wishing to avoid/achieve pregnancy in this cycle:

Anything else of importance in this cycle:

Cycle number: [ ]

Shortest cycle so far: ________ days

Longest cycle so far: ________ days

Where was temperature taken:
Rectum ☐
Vagina ☐
Mouth ☐
Ear ☐

First day of cycle: _____ . _____ . 20 _____   Thermometer: _____________________

Cycle-Day	1	2	3	4	5	6	7	8	9	10	11	12	13	14	15	16	17	18	19	20	21	22	23	24	25	26	27	28	29	30	31	32	33	34	35	36	37	38	39	40
Bleeding																																								
Sex/intercourse (X)																																								
Cervical mucus m = moist s = sticky e = eggwhite																																								
Ovulation (O)																																								

My waking temperature in the morning (also known as basal temperature)

37,5
37,4
37,3
37,2
37,1
37,0
36,9
36,8
36,7
36,6
36,5
36,4
36,3
36,2
36,1

Time of measuring																																								

Cycle-Day	1	2	3	4	5	6	7	8	9	10	11	12	13	14	15	16	17	18	19	20	21	22	23	24	25	26	27	28	29	30	31	32	33	34	35	36	37	38	39	40
Alcohol?																																								
Party, late bedtime?																																								
Ill? Fever?																																								
Breast-feeding? (exclusive/ complementary)																																								
Other notes																																								

Avoiding pregnancy or wanting to achieve one? Some stats on fertility:

Earliest high temperature reading in this cycle on day:

Earliest high temperature reading in all previous cycles including this one:

Deduct 8 to determine the start of your potentially fertile days = the earliest potentially fertile day so far:

Tip: Also record your ovulation day as per your own estimation and gut feeling, as well as the day determined by waking temperature, in the ovulation column. Some women are very aware of their ovaries around the time of ovulation (pulling or stabbing sensation on the right or left, just below the umbilicus). Additionally, around the time of ovulation, your cervical mucus is slippery-stretchy, almost liquid, similar to eggwhite.

Sanitary protection used in this cycle:

Pain levels and/or pain medication used in this cycle:

My experiences with freebleeding in this cycle:

Wishing to avoid/achieve pregnancy in this cycle:

Anything else of importance in this cycle:

Cycle number:

Shortest cycle so far: ________ days

Longest cycle so far: ________ days

Where was temperature taken:
Rectum ☐
Vagina ☐
Mouth ☐
Ear ☐

First day of cycle: _____ . _____ . 20 ____   Thermometer: _________________

Cycle-Day	1	2	3	4	5	6	7	8	9	10	11	12	13	14	15	16	17	18	19	20	21	22	23	24	25	26	27	28	29	30	31	32	33	34	35	36	37	38	39	40
Bleeding																																								
Sex/intercourse (X)																																								
Cervical mucus m = moist s = sticky e = eggwhite																																								
Ovulation (O)																																								

My waking temperature in the morning (also known as basal temperature)

37,5
37,4
37,3
37,2
37,1
37,0
36,9
36,8
36,7
36,6
36,5
36,4
36,3
36,2
36,1

Time of measuring

Cycle-Day	1	2	3	4	5	6	7	8	9	10	11	12	13	14	15	16	17	18	19	20	21	22	23	24	25	26	27	28	29	30	31	32	33	34	35	36	37	38	39	40
Alcohol?																																								
Party, late bedtime?																																								
Ill? Fever?																																								
Breast-feeding? (exclusive/ complementary)																																								
Other notes																																								

Avoiding pregnancy or wanting to achieve one? Some stats on fertility:

Earliest high temperature reading in this cycle on day:

Earliest high temperature reading in all previous cycles including this one:

Deduct 8 to determine the start of your potentially fertile days = the earliest potentially fertile day so far:

Tip: Also record your ovulation day as per your own estimation and gut feeling, as well as the day determined by waking temperature, in the ovulation column. Some women are very aware of their ovaries around the time of ovulation (pulling or stabbing sensation on the right or left, just below the umbilicus). Additionally, around the time of ovulation, your cervical mucus is slippery-stretchy, almost liquid, similar to eggwhite.

Sanitary protection used in this cycle:

Pain levels and/or pain medication used in this cycle:

My experiences with freebleeding in this cycle:

Wishing to avoid/achieve pregnancy in this cycle:

Anything else of importance in this cycle:

Cycle number: [ ]

Shortest cycle so far: ________ days

Longest cycle so far: ________ days

Where was temperature taken:
Rectum ☐
Vagina ☐
Mouth ☐
Ear ☐

First day of cycle: _____ . _____ . 20 _____   Thermometer: _________________

Cycle-Day	1	2	3	4	5	6	7	8	9	10	11	12	13	14	15	16	17	18	19	20	21	22	23	24	25	26	27	28	29	30	31	32	33	34	35	36	37	38	39	40
Bleeding																																								
Sex/intercourse (X)																																								
Cervical mucus m = moist s = sticky e = eggwhite																																								
Ovulation (O)																																								

My waking temperature in the morning (also known as basal temperature)

37,5
37,4
37,3
37,2
37,1
37,0
36,9
36,8
36,7
36,6
36,5
36,4
36,3
36,2
36,1

Time of measuring																																								

Cycle-Day	1	2	3	4	5	6	7	8	9	10	11	12	13	14	15	16	17	18	19	20	21	22	23	24	25	26	27	28	29	30	31	32	33	34	35	36	37	38	39	40
Alcohol?																																								
Party, late bedtime?																																								
Ill? Fever?																																								
Breast-feeding? (exclusive/complementary)																																								
Other notes																																								

Avoiding pregnancy or wanting to achieve one? Some stats on fertility:

Earliest high temperature reading in this cycle on day:

Earliest high temperature reading in all previous cycles including this one:

Deduct 8 to determine the start of your potentially fertile days = the earliest potentially fertile day so far:

Tip: Also record your ovulation day as per your own estimation and gut feeling, as well as the day determined by waking temperature, in the ovulation column. Some women are very aware of their ovaries around the time of ovulation (pulling or stabbing sensation on the right or left, just below the umbilicus). Additionally, around the time of ovulation, your cervical mucus is slippery-stretchy, almost liquid, similar to eggwhite.

Sanitary protection used in this cycle:

Pain levels and/or pain medication used in this cycle:

My experiences with freebleeding in this cycle:

Wishing to avoid/achieve pregnancy in this cycle:

Anything else of importance in this cycle:

Cycle number: [ ]

Shortest cycle so far: ________ days

Longest cycle so far: ________ days

Where was temperature taken:
Rectum ☐
Vagina ☐
Mouth ☐
Ear ☐

First day of cycle: ____ . ____ . 20 ____   Thermometer: _________________

Cycle-Day	1	2	3	4	5	6	7	8	9	10	11	12	13	14	15	16	17	18	19	20	21	22	23	24	25	26	27	28	29	30	31	32	33	34	35	36	37	38	39	40
Bleeding																																								
Sex/intercourse (X)																																								
Cervical mucus m = moist s = sticky e = eggwhite																																								
Ovulation (O)																																								

My waking temperature in the morning (also known as basal temperature)

37,5
37,4
37,3
37,2
37,1
37,0
36,9
36,8
36,7
36,6
36,5
36,4
36,3
36,2
36,1

Time of measuring

Cycle-Day	1	2	3	4	5	6	7	8	9	10	11	12	13	14	15	16	17	18	19	20	21	22	23	24	25	26	27	28	29	30	31	32	33	34	35	36	37	38	39	40
Alcohol?																																								
Party, late bedtime?																																								
Ill? Fever?																																								
Breast-feeding? (exclusive/complementary)																																								
Other notes																																								

Avoiding pregnancy or wanting to achieve one? Some stats on fertility:

Earliest high temperature reading in this cycle on day:

Earliest high temperature reading in all previous cycles including this one:

Deduct 8 to determine the start of your potentially fertile days = the earliest potentially fertile day so far:

Tip: Also record your ovulation day as per your own estimation and gut feeling, as well as the day determined by waking temperature, in the ovulation column. Some women are very aware of their ovaries around the time of ovulation (pulling or stabbing sensation on the right or left, just below the umbilicus). Additionally, around the time of ovulation, your cervical mucus is slippery-stretchy, almost liquid, similar to eggwhite.

Sanitary protection used in this cycle:

Pain levels and/or pain medication used in this cycle:

My experiences with freebleeding in this cycle:

Wishing to avoid/achieve pregnancy in this cycle:

Anything else of importance in this cycle:

Cycle number: ________

Shortest cycle so far: __________ days

Longest cycle so far: __________ days

Where was temperature taken:
Rectum ☐
Vagina ☐
Mouth ☐
Ear ☐

First day of cycle: _____ . _____ . 20 _____   Thermometer: __________________

Cycle-Day	1	2	3	4	5	6	7	8	9	10	11	12	13	14	15	16	17	18	19	20	21	22	23	24	25	26	27	28	29	30	31	32	33	34	35	36	37	38	39	40
Bleeding																																								
Sex/intercourse (X)																																								
Cervical mucus (m = moist, s = sticky, e = eggwhite)																																								
Ovulation (O)																																								

My waking temperature in the morning (also known as basal temperature):

37,5 / 37,4 / 37,3 / 37,2 / 37,1 / **37,0** / 36,9 / 36,8 / 36,7 / 36,6 / 36,5 / 36,4 / 36,3 / 36,2 / 36,1

Time of measuring

Cycle-Day	1	2	3	4	5	6	7	8	9	10	11	12	13	14	15	16	17	18	19	20	21	22	23	24	25	26	27	28	29	30	31	32	33	34	35	36	37	38	39	40
Alcohol?																																								
Party, late bedtime?																																								
Ill? Fever?																																								
Breast-feeding? (exclusive/complementary)																																								
Other notes																																								

Avoiding pregnancy or wanting to achieve one? Some stats on fertility:

Earliest high temperature reading in this cycle on day:

Earliest high temperature reading in all previous cycles including this one:

Deduct 8 to determine the start of your potentially fertile days = the earliest potentially fertile day so far:

Tip: Also record your ovulation day as per your own estimation and gut feeling, as well as the day determined by waking temperature, in the ovulation column. Some women are very aware of their ovaries around the time of ovulation (pulling or stabbing sensation on the right or left, just below the umbilicus). Additionally, around the time of ovulation, your cervical mucus is slippery-stretchy, almost liquid, similar to eggwhite.

Sanitary protection used in this cycle:

Pain levels and/or pain medication used in this cycle:

My experiences with freebleeding in this cycle:

Wishing to avoid/achieve pregnancy in this cycle:

Anything else of importance in this cycle:

$\mathcal{C}ycle\ number:$

Shortest cycle so far: _______ days

Longest cycle so far: _______ days

Where was temperature taken:
Rectum ☐
Vagina ☐
Mouth ☐
Ear ☐

First day of cycle: ____ . ____ . 20 ____   Thermometer: ________________

Cycle-Day	1	2	3	4	5	6	7	8	9	10	11	12	13	14	15	16	17	18	19	20	21	22	23	24	25	26	27	28	29	30	31	32	33	34	35	36	37	38	39	40
Bleeding																																								
Sex/intercourse (X)																																								
Cervical mucus m = moist s = sticky e = eggwhite																																								
Ovulation (O)																																								

My waking temperature in the morning (also known as basal temperature)

37,5
37,4
37,3
37,2
37,1
37,0
36,9
36,8
36,7
36,6
36,5
36,4
36,3
36,2
36,1

Time of measuring

Cycle-Day	1	2	3	4	5	6	7	8	9	10	11	12	13	14	15	16	17	18	19	20	21	22	23	24	25	26	27	28	29	30	31	32	33	34	35	36	37	38	39	40
Alcohol?																																								
Party, late bedtime?																																								
Ill? Fever?																																								
Breast-feeding? (exclusive/ complementary)																																								
Other notes																																								

Avoiding pregnancy or wanting to achieve one? Some stats on fertility:

Earliest high temperature reading in this cycle on day:

Earliest high temperature reading in all previous cycles including this one:

Deduct **8** to determine the start of your potentially fertile days = the earliest potentially fertile day so far:

Tip: Also record your ovulation day as per your own estimation and gut feeling, as well as the day determined by waking temperature, in the ovulation column. Some women are very aware of their ovaries around the time of ovulation (pulling or stabbing sensation on the right or left, just below the umbilicus). Additionally, around the time of ovulation, your cervical mucus is slippery-stretchy, almost liquid, similar to eggwhite.

Sanitary protection used in this cycle:

Pain levels and/or pain medication used in this cycle:

My experiences with freebleeding in this cycle:

Wishing to avoid/achieve pregnancy in this cycle:

Anything else of importance in this cycle:

Cycle number: [ ]

Shortest cycle so far: _________ days

Longest cycle so far: _________ days

Where was temperature taken:
Rectum ☐
Vagina ☐
Mouth ☐
Ear ☐

First day of cycle: _____ . _____ . 20 _____   Thermometer: _____________________

Cycle-Day	1	2	3	4	5	6	7	8	9	10	11	12	13	14	15	16	17	18	19	20	21	22	23	24	25	26	27	28	29	30	31	32	33	34	35	36	37	38	39	40
Bleeding																																								
Sex/intercourse (X)																																								
Cervical mucus **m = moist** **s = sticky** **e = eggwhite**																																								
Ovulation (O)																																								

My waking temperature in the morning (also known as basal temperature)

| | 37,5 |
| 37,4 |
| 37,3 |
| 37,2 |
| 37,1 |
| **37,0** |
| 36,9 |
| 36,8 |
| 36,7 |
| 36,6 |
| 36,5 |
| 36,4 |
| 36,3 |
| 36,2 |
| 36,1 |

Time of measuring

Cycle-Day	1	2	3	4	5	6	7	8	9	10	11	12	13	14	15	16	17	18	19	20	21	22	23	24	25	26	27	28	29	30	31	32	33	34	35	36	37	38	39	40
Alcohol?																																								
Party, late bedtime?																																								
Ill? Fever?																																								
Breastfeeding? (exclusive/ complementary)																																								
Other notes																																								

Avoiding pregnancy or wanting to achieve one? Some stats on fertility:

Earliest high temperature reading in this cycle on day:

Earliest high temperature reading in all previous cycles including this one:

Deduct 8 to determine the **start of** your potentially fertile days = the earliest potentially fertile day so far:

Tip: Also record your **ovulation day** as per your own estimation and gut feeling, as well as the day determined by waking temperature, in the ovulation column. Some women are very aware of their ovaries around the time of ovulation (pulling or stabbing sensation on **the right** or left, just below the umbilicus). Additionally, around the time of ovulation, your cervical mucus is slippery-**stretchy**, almost liquid, similar to eggwhite.

Sanitary protection used in **this cycle:**

Pain levels and/or pain **medication** used in this cycle:

My experiences with **freebleeding** in this cycle:

Wishing to avoid/achieve pregnancy in this cycle:

Anything else of importance in **this cycle:**

Cycle number: [ ]

Shortest cycle so far: ________ days

Longest cycle so far: ________ days

Where was temperature taken:
Rectum ☐
Vagina ☐
Mouth ☐
Ear ☐

First day of cycle: _____ . _____ . 20 _____   Thermometer: _______________

Cycle-Day	1	2	3	4	5	6	7	8	9	10	11	12	13	14	15	16	17	18	19	20	21	22	23	24	25	26	27	28	29	30	31	32	33	34	35	36	37	38	39	40
Bleeding																																								
Sex/intercourse (X)																																								
Cervical mucus m = moist s = sticky e = eggwhite																																								
Ovulation (O)																																								

My waking temperature in the morning (also known as basal temperature)

37,5	
37,4	
37,3	
37,2	
37,1	
37,0	
36,9	
36,8	
36,7	
36,6	
36,5	
36,4	
36,3	
36,2	
36,1	

Time of measuring																																								

Cycle-Day	1	2	3	4	5	6	7	8	9	10	11	12	13	14	15	16	17	18	19	20	21	22	23	24	25	26	27	28	29	30	31	32	33	34	35	36	37	38	39	40
Alcohol?																																								
Party, late bedtime?																																								
Ill? Fever?																																								
Breast-feeding? (exclusive/complementary)																																								
Other notes																																								

Avoiding pregnancy or wanting to achieve one? Some stats on fertility:

Earliest high temperature reading in this cycle on day: ☐☐

Earliest high temperature reading in all previous cycles including this one: ☐☐

Deduct **8** to determine the start of your potentially fertile days = the earliest potentially fertile day so far: ☐☐

Tip: Also record your ovulation day as per your own estimation and gut feeling, as well as the day determined by waking temperature, in the ovulation column. Some women are very aware of their ovaries around the time of ovulation (pulling or stabbing sensation on the right or left, just below the umbilicus). Additionally, around the time of ovulation, your cervical mucus is slippery-stretchy, almost liquid, similar to eggwhite.

Sanitary protection used in this cycle:

Pain levels and/or pain medication used in this cycle:

My experiences with freebleeding in this cycle:

Wishing to avoid/achieve pregnancy in this cycle:

Anything else of importance in this cycle:

Cycle number:

Shortest cycle so far: ________ days

Longest cycle so far: ________ days

Where was temperature taken:
Rectum ☐
Vagina ☐
Mouth ☐
Ear ☐

First day of cycle: _____ . _____ . 20 __________ Thermometer: _________________

Cycle-Day	1	2	3	4	5	6	7	8	9	10	11	12	13	14	15	16	17	18	19	20	21	22	23	24	25	26	27	28	29	30	31	32	33	34	35	36	37	38	39	40
Bleeding																																								
Sex/intercourse (X)																																								
Cervical mucus m = moist s = sticky e = eggwhite																																								
Ovulation (O)																																								

My waking temperature in the morning (also known as basal temperature)

37,5
37,4
37,3
37,2
37,1
37,0
36,9
36,8
36,7
36,6
36,5
36,4
36,3
36,2
36,1

Time of measuring

Cycle-Day	1	2	3	4	5	6	7	8	9	10	11	12	13	14	15	16	17	18	19	20	21	22	23	24	25	26	27	28	29	30	31	32	33	34	35	36	37	38	39	40
Alcohol?																																								
Party, late bedtime?																																								
Ill? Fever?																																								
Breast-feeding? (exclusive/ complementary)																																								
Other notes																																								

Avoiding pregnancy or wanting to achieve one? Some stats on fertility:

Earliest high temperature reading in this cycle on day:

Earliest high temperature reading in all previous cycles including this one:

Deduct 8 to determine the start of your potentially fertile days = the earliest potentially fertile day so far:

Tip: Also record your ovulation day as per your own estimation and gut feeling, as well as the day determined by waking temperature, in the ovulation column. Some women are very aware of their ovaries around the time of ovulation (pulling or stabbing sensation on the right or left, just below the umbilicus). Additionally, around the time of ovulation, your cervical mucus is slippery-stretchy, almost liquid, similar to eggwhite.

Sanitary protection used in this cycle:

Pain levels and/or pain medication used in this cycle:

My experiences with freebleeding in this cycle:

Wishing to avoid/achieve pregnancy in this cycle:

Anything else of importance in this cycle:

Cycle number: [ ]

Shortest cycle so far: ________ days

Longest cycle so far: ________ days

Where was temperature taken:
Rectum ☐
Vagina ☐
Mouth ☐
Ear ☐

First day of cycle: _____ . _____ . 20 ____   Thermometer: _________________

Cycle-Day	1	2	3	4	5	6	7	8	9	10	11	12	13	14	15	16	17	18	19	20	21	22	23	24	25	26	27	28	29	30	31	32	33	34	35	36	37	38	39	40
Bleeding																																								
Sex/intercourse (X)																																								
Cervical mucus m = moist s = sticky e = eggwhite																																								
Ovulation (O)																																								

My waking temperature in the morning (also known as basal temperature)

37,5
37,4
37,3
37,2
37,1
37,0
36,9
36,8
36,7
36,6
36,5
36,4
36,3
36,2
36,1

Time of measuring

Cycle-Day	1	2	3	4	5	6	7	8	9	10	11	12	13	14	15	16	17	18	19	20	21	22	23	24	25	26	27	28	29	30	31	32	33	34	35	36	37	38	39	40
Alcohol?																																								
Party, late bedtime?																																								
Ill? Fever?																																								
Breast-feeding? (exclusive/complementary)																																								
Other notes																																								

Avoiding pregnancy or wanting to achieve one? Some stats on fertility:

Earliest high temperature reading in this cycle on day:

Earliest high temperature reading in all previous cycles including this one:

Deduct 8 to determine the start of your potentially fertile days = the earliest potentially fertile day so far:

Tip: Also record your ovulation day as per your own estimation and gut feeling, as well as the day determined by waking temperature, in the ovulation column. Some women are very aware of their ovaries around the time of ovulation (pulling or stabbing sensation on the right or left, just below the umbilicus). Additionally, around the time of ovulation, your cervical mucus is slippery-stretchy, almost liquid, similar to eggwhite.

Sanitary protection used in this cycle:

Pain levels and/or pain medication used in this cycle:

My experiences with freebleeding in this cycle:

Wishing to avoid/achieve pregnancy in this cycle:

Anything else of importance in this cycle:

Cycle number: [ ]

Shortest cycle so far: _________ days

Longest cycle so far: _________ days

Where was temperature taken:
- Rectum ☐
- Vagina ☐
- Mouth ☐
- Ear ☐

First day of cycle: ______ . ______ . 20 ______   Thermometer: ____________________

Cycle-Day	1	2	3	4	5	6	7	8	9	10	11	12	13	14	15	16	17	18	19	20	21	22	23	24	25	26	27	28	29	30	31	32	33	34	35	36	37	38	39	40
Bleeding																																								
Sex/inter-course (X)																																								
Cervical mucus **m = moist** **s = sticky** **e = eggwhite**																																								
Ovulation (O)																																								

My waking temperature in the morning (also known as basal temperature)

- 37,5
- 37,4
- 37,3
- 37,2
- 37,1
- **37,0**
- 36,9
- 36,8
- 36,7
- 36,6
- 36,5
- 36,4
- 36,3
- 36,2
- 36,1

Time of measuring

Cycle-Day	1	2	3	4	5	6	7	8	9	10	11	12	13	14	15	16	17	18	19	20	21	22	23	24	25	26	27	28	29	30	31	32	33	34	35	36	37	38	39	40
Alcohol?																																								
Party, late bedtime?																																								
Ill? Fever?																																								
Breast-feeding? (exclusive/complementary)																																								
Other notes																																								

Avoiding pregnancy or wanting to achieve one? Some stats on fertility:

Earliest high temperature reading in this cycle on day: ☐ ☐

Earliest high temperature reading in all previous cycles including this one: ☐ ☐

Deduct 8 to determine the start of your potentially fertile days = the earliest potentially fertile day so far: ☐ ☐

Tip: Also record your ovulation day as per your own estimation and gut feeling, as well as the day determined by waking temperature, in the ovulation column. Some women are very aware of their ovaries around the time of ovulation (pulling or stabbing sensation on the right or left, just below the umbilicus). Additionally, around the time of ovulation, your cervical mucus is slippery-stretchy, almost liquid, similar to eggwhite.

Sanitary protection used in this cycle:

Pain levels and/or pain medication used in this cycle:

My experiences with freebleeding in this cycle:

Wishing to avoid/achieve pregnancy in this cycle:

Anything else of importance in this cycle:

Cycle number: [ ]

Shortest cycle so far: ________ days

Longest cycle so far: ________ days

Where was temperature taken:
Rectum ☐
Vagina ☐
Mouth ☐
Ear ☐

First day of cycle: ____ . ____ . 20 ____   Thermometer: ___________________

Cycle-Day	1	2	3	4	5	6	7	8	9	10	11	12	13	14	15	16	17	18	19	20	21	22	23	24	25	26	27	28	29	30	31	32	33	34	35	36	37	38	39	40
Bleeding																																								
Sex/intercourse (X)																																								
Cervical mucus **m = moist** **s = sticky** **e = eggwhite**																																								
Ovulation (O)																																								

My waking temperature in the morning (also known as basal temperature)

37,5
37,4
37,3
37,2
37,1
37,0
36,9
36,8
36,7
36,6
36,5
36,4
36,3
36,2
36,1

Time of measuring

Cycle-Day	1	2	3	4	5	6	7	8	9	10	11	12	13	14	15	16	17	18	19	20	21	22	23	24	25	26	27	28	29	30	31	32	33	34	35	36	37	38	39	40
Alcohol?																																								
Party, late bedtime?																																								
Ill? Fever?																																								
Breast-feeding? (exclusive/complementary)																																								
Other notes																																								

Avoiding pregnancy or wanting to achieve one? Some stats on fertility:

Earliest high temperature reading in this cycle on day:

Earliest high temperature reading in all previous cycles including this one:

Deduct 8 to determine the start of your potentially fertile days = the earliest potentially fertile day so far:

Tip: Also record your ovulation day as per your own estimation and gut feeling, as well as the day determined by waking temperature, in the ovulation column. Some women are very aware of their ovaries around the time of ovulation (pulling or stabbing sensation on the right or left, just below the umbilicus). Additionally, around the time of ovulation, your cervical mucus is slippery-stretchy, almost liquid, similar to eggwhite.

Sanitary protection used in this cycle:

Pain levels and/or pain medication used in this cycle:

My experiences with freebleeding in this cycle:

Wishing to avoid/achieve pregnancy in this cycle:

Anything else of importance in this cycle:

Cycle number:

Shortest cycle so far: _________ days

Longest cycle so far: _________ days

Where was temperature taken:
- Rectum ☐
- Vagina ☐
- Mouth ☐
- Ear ☐

First day of cycle: _____ . _____ . 20 _____   Thermometer: _______________

Cycle-Day	1	2	3	4	5	6	7	8	9	10	11	12	13	14	15	16	17	18	19	20	21	22	23	24	25	26	27	28	29	30	31	32	33	34	35	36	37	38	39	40
Bleeding																																								
Sex/inter-course (X)																																								
Cervical mucus m = moist s = sticky e = eggwhite																																								
Ovulation (O)																																								

My waking temperature in the morning (also known as basal temperature)

| | 37,5 |
| 37,4 |
| 37,3 |
| 37,2 |
| 37,1 |
| **37,0** |
| 36,9 |
| 36,8 |
| 36,7 |
| 36,6 |
| 36,5 |
| 36,4 |
| 36,3 |
| 36,2 |
| 36,1 |

Time of measuring

Cycle-Day	1	2	3	4	5	6	7	8	9	10	11	12	13	14	15	16	17	18	19	20	21	22	23	24	25	26	27	28	29	30	31	32	33	34	35	36	37	38	39	40
Alcohol?																																								
Party, late bedtime?																																								
Ill? Fever?																																								
Breast-feeding? (exclusive/complementary)																																								
Other notes																																								

Avoiding pregnancy or wanting to achieve one? Some stats on fertility:

Earliest high temperature reading in this cycle on day:

Earliest high temperature reading in all previous cycles including this one:

Deduct 8 to determine the start of your potentially fertile days = the earliest potentially fertile day so far:

Tip: Also record your ovulation day as per your own estimation and gut feeling, as well as the day determined by waking temperature, in the ovulation column. Some women are very aware of their ovaries around the time of ovulation (pulling or stabbing sensation on the right or left, just below the umbilicus). Additionally, around the time of ovulation, your cervical mucus is slippery-stretchy, almost liquid, similar to eggwhite.

Sanitary protection used in this cycle:

Pain levels and/or pain medication used in this cycle:

My experiences with freebleeding in this cycle:

Wishing to avoid/achieve pregnancy in this cycle:

Anything else of importance in this cycle:

Cycle number:

Shortest cycle so far: _______ days

Longest cycle so far: _______ days

Where was temperature taken:
Rectum ☐
Vagina ☐
Mouth ☐
Ear ☐

First day of cycle: _____ . _____ . 20 ____   Thermometer: _________________

Cycle-Day	1	2	3	4	5	6	7	8	9	10	11	12	13	14	15	16	17	18	19	20	21	22	23	24	25	26	27	28	29	30	31	32	33	34	35	36	37	38	39	40
Bleeding																																								
Sex/inter-course (X)																																								
Cervical mucus m = moist s = sticky e = eggwhite																																								
Ovulation (O)																																								

My waking temperature in the morning (also known as basal temperature)

	37,5
	37,4
	37,3
	37,2
	37,1
	37,0
	36,9
	36,8
	36,7
	36,6
	36,5
	36,4
	36,3
	36,2
	36,1

Time of measuring

Cycle-Day	1	2	3	4	5	6	7	8	9	10	11	12	13	14	15	16	17	18	19	20	21	22	23	24	25	26	27	28	29	30	31	32	33	34	35	36	37	38	39	40
Alcohol?																																								
Party, late bedtime?																																								
Ill? Fever?																																								
Breast-feeding? (exclusive/complementary)																																								
Other notes																																								

Avoiding pregnancy or wanting to achieve one? Some stats on fertility:

Earliest high temperature reading in this cycle on day:

Earliest high temperature reading in all previous cycles including this one:

Deduct 8 to determine the start of your potentially fertile days = the earliest potentially fertile day so far:

Tip: Also record your ovulation day as per your own estimation and gut feeling, as well as the day determined by waking temperature, in the ovulation column. Some women are very aware of their ovaries around the time of ovulation (pulling or stabbing sensation on the right or left, just below the umbilicus). Additionally, around the time of ovulation, your cervical mucus is slippery-stretchy, almost liquid, similar to eggwhite.

Sanitary protection used in this cycle:

Pain levels and/or pain medication used in this cycle:

My experiences with freebleeding in this cycle:

Wishing to avoid/achieve pregnancy in this cycle:

Anything else of importance in this cycle:

Cycle number: [ ]

Shortest cycle so far: _________ days

Longest cycle so far: _________ days

Where was temperature taken:
Rectum ☐
Vagina ☐
Mouth ☐
Ear ☐

First day of cycle: _____ . _____ . 20 _____   Thermometer: ____________________

Cycle-Day	1	2	3	4	5	6	7	8	9	10	11	12	13	14	15	16	17	18	19	20	21	22	23	24	25	26	27	28	29	30	31	32	33	34	35	36	37	38	39	40
Bleeding																																								
Sex/intercourse (X)																																								
Cervical mucus m = moist s = sticky e = eggwhite																																								
Ovulation (O)																																								

My waking temperature in the morning (also known as basal temperature)

| | 37,5 |
| 37,4 |
| 37,3 |
| 37,2 |
| 37,1 |
| **37,0** |
| 36,9 |
| 36,8 |
| 36,7 |
| 36,6 |
| 36,5 |
| 36,4 |
| 36,3 |
| 36,2 |
| 36,1 |

Time of measuring

Cycle-Day	1	2	3	4	5	6	7	8	9	10	11	12	13	14	15	16	17	18	19	20	21	22	23	24	25	26	27	28	29	30	31	32	33	34	35	36	37	38	39	40
Alcohol?																																								
Party, late bedtime?																																								
Ill? Fever?																																								
Breast-feeding? (exclusive/complementary)																																								
Other notes																																								

Avoiding pregnancy or wanting to achieve one? Some stats on fertility:

Earliest high temperature reading in this cycle on day:

Earliest high temperature reading in all previous cycles including this one:

Deduct 8 to determine the start of your potentially fertile days = the earliest potentially fertile day so far:

Tip: Also record your ovulation day as per your own estimation and gut feeling, as well as the day determined by waking temperature, in the ovulation column. Some women are very aware of their ovaries around the time of ovulation (pulling or stabbing sensation on the right or left, just below the umbilicus). Additionally, around the time of ovulation, your cervical mucus is slippery-stretchy, almost liquid, similar to eggwhite.

Sanitary protection used in this cycle:

Pain levels and/or pain medication used in this cycle:

My experiences with freebleeding in this cycle:

Wishing to avoid/achieve pregnancy in this cycle:

Anything else of importance in this cycle:

Cycle number:

Shortest cycle so far: _________ days

Longest cycle so far: _________ days

Where was temperature taken:
Rectum ☐
Vagina ☐
Mouth ☐
Ear ☐

First day of cycle: _____ . _____ . 20 _____   Thermometer: _________________

Cycle-Day	1	2	3	4	5	6	7	8	9	10	11	12	13	14	15	16	17	18	19	20	21	22	23	24	25	26	27	28	29	30	31	32	33	34	35	36	37	38	39	40
Bleeding																																								
Sex/intercourse (X)																																								
Cervical mucus m = moist s = sticky e = eggwhite																																								
Ovulation (O)																																								

My waking temperature in the morning (also known as basal temperature)

37,5
37,4
37,3
37,2
37,1
37,0
36,9
36,8
36,7
36,6
36,5
36,4
36,3
36,2
36,1

Time of measuring																																								

Cycle-Day	1	2	3	4	5	6	7	8	9	10	11	12	13	14	15	16	17	18	19	20	21	22	23	24	25	26	27	28	29	30	31	32	33	34	35	36	37	38	39	40
Alcohol?																																								
Party, late bedtime?																																								
Ill? Fever?																																								
Breast-feeding? (exclusive/ complementary)																																								
Other notes																																								

Avoiding pregnancy or wanting to achieve one? Some stats on fertility:

Earliest high temperature reading in this cycle on day:

Earliest high temperature reading in all previous cycles including this one:

Deduct 8 to determine the start of your potentially fertile days = the earliest potentially fertile day so far:

Tip: Also record your ovulation day as per your own estimation and gut feeling, as well as the day determined by waking temperature, in the ovulation column. Some women are very aware of their ovaries around the time of ovulation (pulling or stabbing sensation on the right or left, just below the umbilicus). Additionally, around the time of ovulation, your cervical mucus is slippery-stretchy, almost liquid, similar to eggwhite.

Sanitary protection used in this cycle:

Pain levels and/or pain medication used in this cycle:

My experiences with freebleeding in this cycle:

Wishing to avoid/achieve pregnancy in this cycle:

Anything else of importance in this cycle:

Cycle number: [ ]

Shortest cycle so far: _________ days

Longest cycle so far: _________ days

Where was temperature taken:
Rectum ☐
Vagina ☐
Mouth ☐
Ear ☐

First day of cycle: _____ . _____ . 20 _____   Thermometer: _________________

Cycle-Day	1	2	3	4	5	6	7	8	9	10	11	12	13	14	15	16	17	18	19	20	21	22	23	24	25	26	27	28	29	30	31	32	33	34	35	36	37	38	39	40
Bleeding																																								
Sex/intercourse (X)																																								
Cervical mucus **m = moist** **s = sticky** **e = eggwhite**																																								
Ovulation (O)																																								

My waking temperature in the morning (also known as basal temperature):

- 37,5
- 37,4
- 37,3
- 37,2
- 37,1
- **37,0**
- 36,9
- 36,8
- 36,7
- 36,6
- 36,5
- 36,4
- 36,3
- 36,2
- 36,1

Time of measuring

Cycle-Day	1	2	3	4	5	6	7	8	9	10	11	12	13	14	15	16	17	18	19	20	21	22	23	24	25	26	27	28	29	30	31	32	33	34	35	36	37	38	39	40
Alcohol?																																								
Party, late bedtime?																																								
Ill? Fever?																																								
Breast-feeding? (exclusive/complementary)																																								
Other notes																																								

Avoiding pregnancy or wanting to achieve one? Some stats on fertility:

Earliest high temperature reading in this cycle on day:

Earliest high temperature reading in all previous cycles including this one:

Deduct 8 to determine the start of your potentially fertile days = the earliest potentially fertile day so far:

Tip: Also record your ovulation day as per your own estimation and gut feeling, as well as the day determined by waking temperature, in the ovulation column. Some women are very aware of their ovaries around the time of ovulation (pulling or stabbing sensation on the right or left, just below the umbilicus). Additionally, around the time of ovulation, your cervical mucus is slippery-stretchy, almost liquid, similar to eggwhite.

Sanitary protection used in this cycle:

Pain levels and/or pain medication used in this cycle:

My experiences with freebleeding in this cycle:

Wishing to avoid/achieve pregnancy in this cycle:

Anything else of importance in this cycle:

Cycle-Day	1	2	3	4	5	6	7	8	9	10	11	12	13	14	15	16	17	18	19	20	21	22	23	24	25	26	27	28	29	30	31	32	33	34	35	36	37	38	39	40
Bleeding																																								
Sex/intercourse (X)																																								
Cervical mucus (m = moist, s = sticky, e = eggwhite)																																								
Ovulation (O)																																								

My waking temperature in the morning (also known as basal temperature):

37,5
37,4
37,3
37,2
37,1
37,0
36,9
36,8
36,7
36,6
36,5
36,4
36,3
36,2
36,1

Time of measuring																																								

Cycle-Day	1	2	3	4	5	6	7	8	9	10	11	12	13	14	15	16	17	18	19	20	21	22	23	24	25	26	27	28	29	30	31	32	33	34	35	36	37	38	39	40
Alcohol?																																								
Party, late bedtime?																																								
Ill? Fever?																																								
Breast-feeding? (exclusive/complementary)																																								
Other notes																																								

Avoiding pregnancy or wanting to achieve one? Some stats on fertility:

Earliest high temperature reading in this cycle on day:

Earliest high temperature reading in all previous cycles including this one:

Deduct 8 to determine the start of your potentially fertile days = the earliest potentially fertile day so far:

Tip: Also record your ovulation day as per your own estimation and gut feeling, as well as the day determined by waking temperature, in the ovulation column. Some women are very aware of their ovaries around the time of ovulation (pulling or stabbing sensation on the right or left, just below the umbilicus). Additionally, around the time of ovulation, your cervical mucus is slippery-stretchy, almost liquid, similar to eggwhite.

Sanitary protection used in this cycle:

Pain levels and/or pain medication used in this cycle:

My experiences with freebleeding in this cycle:

Wishing to avoid/achieve pregnancy in this cycle:

Anything else of importance in this cycle:

Cycle number: [ ]

Shortest cycle so far: _________ days

Longest cycle so far: _________ days

Where was temperature taken:
Rectum ☐
Vagina ☐
Mouth ☐
Ear ☐

First day of cycle: _____ . _____ . 20 _____   Thermometer: _____________________

Cycle-Day	1	2	3	4	5	6	7	8	9	10	11	12	13	14	15	16	17	18	19	20	21	22	23	24	25	26	27	28	29	30	31	32	33	34	35	36	37	38	39	40
Bleeding																																								
Sex/inter-course (X)																																								
Cervical mucus m = moist s = sticky e = eggwhite																																								
Ovulation (O)																																								

My waking temperature in the morning (also known as basal temperature)

37,5
37,4
37,3
37,2
37,1
37,0
36,9
36,8
36,7
36,6
36,5
36,4
36,3
36,2
36,1

Time of measuring																																								

Cycle-Day	1	2	3	4	5	6	7	8	9	10	11	12	13	14	15	16	17	18	19	20	21	22	23	24	25	26	27	28	29	30	31	32	33	34	35	36	37	38	39	40
Alcohol?																																								
Party, late bedtime?																																								
Ill? Fever?																																								
Breast-feeding? (exclusive/complemen-tary)																																								
Other notes																																								

Avoiding pregnancy or wanting to achieve one? Some stats on fertility:

Earliest high temperature reading in this cycle on day:

Earliest high temperature reading in all previous cycles including this one:

Deduct 8 to determine the **start of** your potentially fertile days = the earliest potentially fertile day so far:

Tip: Also record your ovulation day as per your own estimation and gut feeling, as well as the day determined by waking temperature, in the ovulation column. Some women are very aware of their ovaries around the time of ovulation (pulling or stabbing sensation on the right or left, just below the umbilicus). Additionally, around the time of ovulation, your cervical mucus is slippery-stretchy, almost liquid, similar to eggwhite.

Sanitary protection used in this cycle:

Pain levels and/or pain medication used in this cycle:

My experiences with freebleeding in this cycle:

Wishing to avoid/achieve pregnancy in this cycle:

Anything else of importance in this cycle:

Cycle number: [ ]

Shortest cycle so far: ________ days

Longest cycle so far: ________ days

Where was temperature taken:
Rectum ☐
Vagina ☐
Mouth ☐
Ear ☐

First day of cycle: _____ . _____ . 20 ____   Thermometer: ___________________

Cycle-Day	1	2	3	4	5	6	7	8	9	10	11	12	13	14	15	16	17	18	19	20	21	22	23	24	25	26	27	28	29	30	31	32	33	34	35	36	37	38	39	40
Bleeding																																								
Sex/intercourse (X)																																								
Cervical mucus m = moist s = sticky e = eggwhite																																								
Ovulation (O)																																								

My waking temperature in the morning (also known as basal temperature)

37,5
37,4
37,3
37,2
37,1
37,0
36,9
36,8
36,7
36,6
36,5
36,4
36,3
36,2
36,1

Time of measuring

Cycle-Day	1	2	3	4	5	6	7	8	9	10	11	12	13	14	15	16	17	18	19	20	21	22	23	24	25	26	27	28	29	30	31	32	33	34	35	36	37	38	39	40
Alcohol?																																								
Party, late bedtime?																																								
Ill? Fever?																																								
Breast-feeding? (exclusive/complementary)																																								
Other notes																																								

Avoiding pregnancy or wanting to achieve one? Some stats on fertility:

Earliest high temperature reading in this cycle on day:

Earliest high temperature reading in all previous cycles including this one:

Deduct 8 to determine the start of your potentially fertile days = the earliest potentially fertile day so far:

Tip: Also record your ovulation day as per your own estimation and gut feeling, as well as the day determined by waking temperature, in the ovulation column. Some women are very aware of their ovaries around the time of ovulation (pulling or stabbing sensation on the right or left, just below the umbilicus). Additionally, around the time of ovulation, your cervical mucus is slippery-stretchy, almost liquid, similar to eggwhite.

Sanitary protection used in this cycle:

Pain levels and/or pain medication used in this cycle:

My experiences with freebleeding in this cycle:

Wishing to avoid/achieve pregnancy in this cycle:

Anything else of importance in this cycle:

Cycle number: ☐

Shortest cycle so far: _________ days

Longest cycle so far: _________ days

Where was temperature taken:
Rectum ☐
Vagina ☐
Mouth ☐
Ear ☐

First day of cycle: _____ . _____ . 20 _____   Thermometer: _______________

Cycle-Day	1	2	3	4	5	6	7	8	9	10	11	12	13	14	15	16	17	18	19	20	21	22	23	24	25	26	27	28	29	30	31	32	33	34	35	36	37	38	39	40
Bleeding																																								
Sex/intercourse (X)																																								
Cervical mucus — m = moist, s = sticky, e = eggwhite																																								
Ovulation (O)																																								

My waking temperature in the morning (also known as basal temperature)

°C	1	2	3	4	5	6	7	8	9	10	11	12	13	14	15	16	17	18	19	20	21	22	23	24	25	26	27	28	29	30	31	32	33	34	35	36	37	38	39	40
37,5																																								
37,4																																								
37,3																																								
37,2																																								
37,1																																								
37,0																																								
36,9																																								
36,8																																								
36,7																																								
36,6																																								
36,5																																								
36,4																																								
36,3																																								
36,2																																								
36,1																																								

Time of measuring																																								

Cycle-Day	1	2	3	4	5	6	7	8	9	10	11	12	13	14	15	16	17	18	19	20	21	22	23	24	25	26	27	28	29	30	31	32	33	34	35	36	37	38	39	40
Alcohol?																																								
Party, late bedtime?																																								
Ill? Fever?																																								
Breast-feeding? (exclusive/complementary)																																								
Other notes																																								

Avoiding pregnancy or wanting to achieve one? Some stats on fertility:

Earliest high temperature reading in this cycle on day:

Earliest high temperature reading in all previous cycles including this one:

Deduct 8 to determine the start of your potentially fertile days = the earliest potentially fertile day so far:

Tip: Also record your ovulation day as per your own estimation and gut feeling, as well as the day determined by waking temperature, in the ovulation column. Some women are very aware of their ovaries around the time of ovulation (pulling or stabbing sensation on the right or left, just below the umbilicus). Additionally, around the time of ovulation, your cervical mucus is slippery-stretchy, almost liquid, similar to eggwhite.

Sanitary protection used in this cycle:

Pain levels and/or pain medication used in this cycle:

My experiences with freebleeding in this cycle:

Wishing to avoid/achieve pregnancy in this cycle:

Anything else of importance in this cycle:

Cycle number: ☐

Shortest cycle so far: ________ days

Longest cycle so far: ________ days

Where was temperature taken:
Rectum ☐
Vagina ☐
Mouth ☐
Ear ☐

First day of cycle: _____ . _____ . 20 _____   Thermometer: _________________

Cycle-Day	1	2	3	4	5	6	7	8	9	10	11	12	13	14	15	16	17	18	19	20	21	22	23	24	25	26	27	28	29	30	31	32	33	34	35	36	37	38	39	40
Bleeding																																								
Sex/intercourse (X)																																								
Cervical mucus (m = moist, s = sticky, e = eggwhite)																																								
Ovulation (O)																																								

My waking temperature in the morning (also known as basal temperature)

| | 37,5 |
| 37,4 |
| 37,3 |
| 37,2 |
| 37,1 |
| **37,0** |
| 36,9 |
| 36,8 |
| 36,7 |
| 36,6 |
| 36,5 |
| 36,4 |
| 36,3 |
| 36,2 |
| 36,1 |

Time of measuring

Cycle-Day	1	2	3	4	5	6	7	8	9	10	11	12	13	14	15	16	17	18	19	20	21	22	23	24	25	26	27	28	29	30	31	32	33	34	35	36	37	38	39	40
Alcohol?																																								
Party, late bedtime?																																								
Ill? Fever?																																								
Breast-feeding? (exclusive/complementary)																																								
Other notes																																								

Avoiding pregnancy or wanting to achieve one? Some stats on fertility:

Earliest high temperature reading in this cycle on day:

Earliest high temperature reading in all previous cycles including this one:

Deduct 8 to determine the start of your potentially fertile days = the earliest potentially fertile day so far:

Tip: Also record your ovulation day as per your own estimation and gut feeling, as well as the day determined by waking temperature, in the ovulation column. Some women are very aware of their ovaries around the time of ovulation (pulling or stabbing sensation on the right or left, just below the umbilicus). Additionally, around the time of ovulation, your cervical mucus is slippery-stretchy, almost liquid, similar to eggwhite.

Sanitary protection used in this cycle:

Pain levels and/or pain medication used in this cycle:

My experiences with freebleeding in this cycle:

Wishing to avoid/achieve pregnancy in this cycle:

Anything else of importance in this cycle:

Cycle number: [ ]

Shortest cycle so far: ________ days

Longest cycle so far: ________ days

Where was temperature taken:
Rectum ☐
Vagina ☐
Mouth ☐
Ear ☐

First day of cycle: ____ . ____ . 20 ____   Thermometer: _________________

Cycle-Day	1	2	3	4	5	6	7	8	9	10	11	12	13	14	15	16	17	18	19	20	21	22	23	24	25	26	27	28	29	30	31	32	33	34	35	36	37	38	39	40
Bleeding																																								
Sex/intercourse (X)																																								
Cervical mucus m = moist s = sticky e = eggwhite																																								
Ovulation (O)																																								

My waking temperature in the morning (also known as basal temperature)

37,5
37,4
37,3
37,2
37,1
37,0
36,9
36,8
36,7
36,6
36,5
36,4
36,3
36,2
36,1

| Time of measuring | | | | | | | | | | | | | | | | | | | | | | | | | | | | | | | | | | | | | | | | |

Cycle-Day	1	2	3	4	5	6	7	8	9	10	11	12	13	14	15	16	17	18	19	20	21	22	23	24	25	26	27	28	29	30	31	32	33	34	35	36	37	38	39	40
Alcohol?																																								
Party, late bedtime?																																								
Ill? Fever?																																								
Breast-feeding? (exclusive/ complementary)																																								
Other notes																																								

Avoiding pregnancy or wanting to achieve one? Some stats on fertility:

Earliest high temperature reading in this cycle on day:

Earliest high temperature reading in all previous cycles including this one:

Deduct 8 to determine the start of your potentially fertile days = the earliest potentially fertile day so far:

Tip: Also record your ovulation day as per your own estimation and gut feeling, as well as the day determined by waking temperature, in the ovulation column. Some women are very aware of their ovaries around the time of ovulation (pulling or stabbing sensation on the right or left, just below the umbilicus). Additionally, around the time of ovulation, your cervical mucus is slippery-stretchy, almost liquid, similar to eggwhite.

Sanitary protection used in this cycle:

Pain levels and/or pain medication used in this cycle:

My experiences with freebleeding in this cycle:

Wishing to avoid/achieve pregnancy in this cycle:

Anything else of importance in this cycle:

Cycle number: [ ]

Shortest cycle so far: _________ days

Longest cycle so far: _________ days

Where was temperature taken:
Rectum ☐
Vagina ☐
Mouth ☐
Ear ☐

First day of cycle: _____ . _____ . 20 _____   Thermometer: _________________

Cycle-Day	1	2	3	4	5	6	7	8	9	10	11	12	13	14	15	16	17	18	19	20	21	22	23	24	25	26	27	28	29	30	31	32	33	34	35	36	37	38	39	40
Bleeding																																								
Sex/inter-course (X)																																								
Cervical mucus **m = moist s = sticky e = eggwhite**																																								
Ovulation (O)																																								

My waking temperature in the morning (also known as basal temperature)

| | 37,5 |
| 37,4 |
| 37,3 |
| 37,2 |
| 37,1 |
| **37,0** |
| 36,9 |
| 36,8 |
| 36,7 |
| 36,6 |
| 36,5 |
| 36,4 |
| 36,3 |
| 36,2 |
| 36,1 |

| Time of measuring | | | | | | | | | | | | | | | | | | | | | | | | | | | | | | | | | | | | | | | | |

Cycle-Day	1	2	3	4	5	6	7	8	9	10	11	12	13	14	15	16	17	18	19	20	21	22	23	24	25	26	27	28	29	30	31	32	33	34	35	36	37	38	39	40
Alcohol?																																								
Party, late bedtime?																																								
Ill? Fever?																																								
Breast-feeding? (exclusive/ complementary)																																								
Other notes																																								

Avoiding pregnancy or wanting to achieve one? Some stats on fertility:

Earliest high temperature reading in this cycle on day:

Earliest high temperature reading in all previous cycles including this one:

Deduct 8 to determine the start of your potentially fertile days = the earliest potentially fertile day so far:

Tip: Also record your ovulation day as per your own estimation and gut feeling, as well as the day determined by waking temperature, in the ovulation column. Some women are very aware of their ovaries around the time of ovulation (pulling or stabbing sensation on the right or left, just below the umbilicus). Additionally, around the time of ovulation, your cervical mucus is slippery-stretchy, almost liquid, similar to eggwhite.

Sanitary protection used in this cycle:

Pain levels and/or pain medication used in this cycle:

My experiences with freebleeding in this cycle:

Wishing to avoid/achieve pregnancy in this cycle:

Anything else of importance in this cycle:

Cycle number:

Shortest cycle so far: ________ days

Longest cycle so far: ________ days

Where was temperature taken:
Rectum ☐
Vagina ☐
Mouth ☐
Ear ☐

First day of cycle: _____ . _____ . 20 ____ Thermometer: __________________

Cycle-Day	1	2	3	4	5	6	7	8	9	10	11	12	13	14	15	16	17	18	19	20	21	22	23	24	25	26	27	28	29	30	31	32	33	34	35	36	37	38	39	40
Bleeding																																								
Sex/intercourse (X)																																								
Cervical mucus (m = moist, s = sticky, e = eggwhite)																																								
Ovulation (O)																																								

My waking temperature in the morning (also known as basal temperature):

37,5 / 37,4 / 37,3 / 37,2 / 37,1 / **37,0** / 36,9 / 36,8 / 36,7 / 36,6 / 36,5 / 36,4 / 36,3 / 36,2 / 36,1

Time of measuring

Cycle-Day	1	2	3	4	5	6	7	8	9	10	11	12	13	14	15	16	17	18	19	20	21	22	23	24	25	26	27	28	29	30	31	32	33	34	35	36	37	38	39	40
Alcohol?																																								
Party, late bedtime?																																								
Ill? Fever?																																								
Breastfeeding? (exclusive/complementary)																																								
Other notes																																								

Avoiding pregnancy or wanting to achieve one? Some stats on fertility:

Earliest high temperature reading in this cycle on day:

Earliest high temperature reading in all previous cycles including this one:

Deduct 8 to determine the start of your potentially fertile days = the earliest potentially fertile day so far:

Tip: Also record your ovulation day as per your own estimation and gut feeling, as well the day determined by waking temperature, in the ovulation column. Some women are very aware of their ovaries around the time of ovulation (pulling or stabbing sensation on the right or left, just below the umbilicus). Additionally, around the time of ovulation, your cervical mucus is slippery-stretchy, almost liquid, similar to eggwhite.

Sanitary protection used in this cycle:

Pain levels and/or pain medication used in this cycle:

My experiences with freebleeding in this cycle:

Wishing to avoid/achieve pregnancy in this cycle:

Anything else of importance in this cycle:

Cycle number: [ ]

Shortest cycle so far: _______ days

Longest cycle so far: _______ days

Where was temperature taken:
Rectum ☐
Vagina ☐
Mouth ☐
Ear ☐

First day of cycle: ____ . ____ . 20____   Thermometer: _______________

Cycle-Day	1	2	3	4	5	6	7	8	9	10	11	12	13	14	15	16	17	18	19	20	21	22	23	24	25	26	27	28	29	30	31	32	33	34	35	36	37	38	39	40
Bleeding																																								
Sex/intercourse (X)																																								
Cervical mucus m = moist s = sticky e = eggwhite																																								
Ovulation (O)																																								

My waking temperature in the morning (also known as basal temperature)

37,5
37,4
37,3
37,2
37,1
37,0
36,9
36,8
36,7
36,6
36,5
36,4
36,3
36,2
36,1

Time of measuring

Cycle-Day	1	2	3	4	5	6	7	8	9	10	11	12	13	14	15	16	17	18	19	20	21	22	23	24	25	26	27	28	29	30	31	32	33	34	35	36	37	38	39	40
Alcohol?																																								
Party, late bedtime?																																								
Ill? Fever?																																								
Breast-feeding? (exclusive/complementary)																																								
Other notes																																								

Avoiding pregnancy or wanting to achieve one? Some stats on fertility:

Earliest high temperature reading in this cycle on day:

Earliest high temperature reading in all previous cycles including this one:

Deduct 8 to determine the start of your potentially fertile days = the earliest potentially fertile day so far:

Tip: Also record your ovulation day as per your own estimation and gut feeling, as well as the day determined by waking temperature, in the ovulation column. Some women are very aware of their ovaries around the time of ovulation (pulling or stabbing sensation on the right or left, just below the umbilicus). Additionally, around the time of ovulation, your cervical mucus is slippery-stretchy, almost liquid, similar to eggwhite.

Sanitary protection used in this cycle:

Pain levels and/or pain medication used in this cycle:

My experiences with freebleeding in this cycle:

Wishing to avoid/achieve pregnancy in this cycle:

Anything else of importance in this cycle:

Cycle number: [ ]

Shortest cycle so far: _________ days

Longest cycle so far: _________ days

Where was temperature taken:
Rectum ☐
Vagina ☐
Mouth ☐
Ear ☐

First day of cycle: _____ . _____ . 20 _____   Thermometer: ____________________

Cycle-Day	1	2	3	4	5	6	7	8	9	10	11	12	13	14	15	16	17	18	19	20	21	22	23	24	25	26	27	28	29	30	31	32	33	34	35	36	37	38	39	40
Bleeding																																								
Sex/intercourse (X)																																								
Cervical mucus m = moist s = sticky e = eggwhite																																								
Ovulation (O)																																								

My waking temperature in the morning (also known as basal temperature)

	37,5
	37,4
	37,3
	37,2
	37,1
	37,0
	36,9
	36,8
	36,7
	36,6
	36,5
	36,4
	36,3
	36,2
	36,1

Time of measuring

Cycle-Day	1	2	3	4	5	6	7	8	9	10	11	12	13	14	15	16	17	18	19	20	21	22	23	24	25	26	27	28	29	30	31	32	33	34	35	36	37	38	39	40
Alcohol?																																								
Party, late bedtime?																																								
Ill? Fever?																																								
Breast-feeding? (exclusive/complementary)																																								
Other notes																																								

Avoiding pregnancy or wanting to achieve one? Some stats on fertility:

Earliest high temperature reading in this cycle on day:

Earliest high temperature reading in all previous cycles including this one:

Deduct 8 to determine the start of your potentially fertile days = the earliest potentially fertile day so far:

Tip: Also record your ovulation day as per your own estimation and gut feeling, as well as the day determined by waking temperature, in the ovulation column. Some women are very aware of their ovaries around the time of ovulation (pulling or stabbing sensation on the right or left, just below the umbilicus). Additionally, around the time of ovulation, your cervical mucus is slippery-stretchy, almost liquid, similar to eggwhite.

Sanitary protection used in this cycle:

Pain levels and/or pain medication used in this cycle:

My experiences with freebleeding in this cycle:

Wishing to avoid/achieve pregnancy in this cycle:

Anything else of importance in this cycle:

Cycle number: [ ]

Shortest cycle so far: _________ days

Longest cycle so far: _________ days

Where was temperature taken:
Rectum ☐
Vagina ☐
Mouth ☐
Ear ☐

First day of cycle: _____ . _____ . 20 _____   Thermometer: _________________

Cycle-Day	1	2	3	4	5	6	7	8	9	10	11	12	13	14	15	16	17	18	19	20	21	22	23	24	25	26	27	28	29	30	31	32	33	34	35	36	37	38	39	40
Bleeding																																								
Sex/intercourse (X)																																								
Cervical mucus m = moist s = sticky e = eggwhite																																								
Ovulation (O)																																								

My waking temperature in the morning (also known as basal temperature)

°C																																								
37,5																																								
37,4																																								
37,3																																								
37,2																																								
37,1																																								
37,0																																								
36,9																																								
36,8																																								
36,7																																								
36,6																																								
36,5																																								
36,4																																								
36,3																																								
36,2																																								
36,1																																								
Time of measuring																																								

Cycle-Day	1	2	3	4	5	6	7	8	9	10	11	12	13	14	15	16	17	18	19	20	21	22	23	24	25	26	27	28	29	30	31	32	33	34	35	36	37	38	39	40
Alcohol?																																								
Party, late bedtime?																																								
Ill? Fever?																																								
Breastfeeding? (exclusive/ complementary)																																								
Other notes																																								

Avoiding pregnancy or wanting to achieve one? Some stats on fertility:

Earliest high temperature reading in this cycle on day:

Earliest high temperature reading in all previous cycles including this one:

Deduct 8 to determine the start of your potentially fertile days = the earliest potentially fertile day so far:

Tip: Also record your ovulation day as per your own estimation and gut feeling, as well as the day determined by waking temperature, in the ovulation column. Some women are very aware of their ovaries around the time of ovulation (pulling or stabbing sensation on the right or left, just below the umbilicus). Additionally, around the time of ovulation, your cervical mucus is slippery-stretchy, almost liquid, similar to eggwhite.

Sanitary protection used in this cycle:

Pain levels and/or pain medication used in this cycle:

My experiences with freebleeding in this cycle:

Wishing to avoid/achieve pregnancy in this cycle:

Anything else of importance in this cycle:

Cycle number: [　]

Shortest cycle so far: _________ days

Longest cycle so far: _________ days

Where was temperature taken:
Rectum ☐
Vagina ☐
Mouth ☐
Ear ☐

First day of cycle: _____ . _____ . 20 _____   Thermometer: _________________

Cycle-Day	1	2	3	4	5	6	7	8	9	10	11	12	13	14	15	16	17	18	19	20	21	22	23	24	25	26	27	28	29	30	31	32	33	34	35	36	37	38	39	40
Bleeding																																								
Sex/intercourse (X)																																								
Cervical mucus m = moist s = sticky e = eggwhite																																								
Ovulation (O)																																								

My waking temperature in the morning (also known as basal temperature)

	37,5
	37,4
	37,3
	37,2
	37,1
	37,0
	36,9
	36,8
	36,7
	36,6
	36,5
	36,4
	36,3
	36,2
	36,1

Time of measuring

Cycle-Day	1	2	3	4	5	6	7	8	9	10	11	12	13	14	15	16	17	18	19	20	21	22	23	24	25	26	27	28	29	30	31	32	33	34	35	36	37	38	39	40
Alcohol?																																								
Party, late bedtime?																																								
Ill? Fever?																																								
Breast-feeding? (exclusive/complementary)																																								
Other notes																																								

Avoiding pregnancy or wanting to achieve one? Some stats on fertility:

Earliest high temperature reading in this cycle on day:

Earliest high temperature reading in all previous cycles including this one:

Deduct 8 to determine the start of your potentially fertile days = the earliest potentially fertile day so far:

Tip: Also record your ovulation day as per your own estimation and gut feeling, as well as the day determined by waking temperature, in the ovulation column. Some women are very aware of their ovaries around the time of ovulation (pulling or stabbing sensation on the right or left, just below the umbilicus). Additionally, around the time of ovulation, your cervical mucus is slippery-stretchy, almost liquid, similar to eggwhite.

Sanitary protection used in this cycle:

Pain levels and/or pain medication used in this cycle:

My experiences with freebleeding in this cycle:

Wishing to avoid/achieve pregnancy in this cycle:

Anything else of importance in this cycle:

Cycle number: [ ]

Shortest cycle so far: _______ days

Longest cycle so far: _______ days

Where was temperature taken:
Rectum ☐
Vagina ☐
Mouth ☐
Ear ☐

First day of cycle: _____ . _____ . 20 _____   Thermometer: _______________

Cycle-Day	1	2	3	4	5	6	7	8	9	10	11	12	13	14	15	16	17	18	19	20	21	22	23	24	25	26	27	28	29	30	31	32	33	34	35	36	37	38	39	40
Bleeding																																								
Sex/intercourse (X)																																								
Cervical mucus m = moist s = sticky e = eggwhite																																								
Ovulation (O)																																								

My waking temperature in the morning (also known as basal temperature)

37,5
37,4
37,3
37,2
37,1
37,0
36,9
36,8
36,7
36,6
36,5
36,4
36,3
36,2
36,1

Time of measuring

Cycle-Day	1	2	3	4	5	6	7	8	9	10	11	12	13	14	15	16	17	18	19	20	21	22	23	24	25	26	27	28	29	30	31	32	33	34	35	36	37	38	39	40
Alcohol?																																								
Party, late bedtime?																																								
Ill? Fever?																																								
Breast-feeding? (exclusive/complementary)																																								
Other notes																																								

Avoiding pregnancy or wanting to achieve one? Some stats on fertility:

Earliest high temperature reading in this cycle on day:

Earliest high temperature reading in all previous cycles including this one:

Deduct 8 to determine the start of your potentially fertile days = the earliest potentially fertile day so far:

Tip: Also record your ovulation day as per your own estimation and gut feeling, as well as the day determined by waking temperature, in the ovulation column. Some women are very aware of their ovaries around the time of ovulation (pulling or stabbing sensation on the right or left, just below the umbilicus). Additionally, around the time of ovulation, your cervical mucus is slippery-stretchy, almost liquid, similar to eggwhite.

Sanitary protection used in this cycle:

Pain levels and/or pain medication used in this cycle:

My experiences with freebleeding in this cycle:

Wishing to avoid/achieve pregnancy in this cycle:

Anything else of importance in this cycle:

Cycle number: ☐

Shortest cycle so far: _________ days

Longest cycle so far: _________ days

Where was temperature taken:
- Rectum ☐
- Vagina ☐
- Mouth ☐
- Ear ☐

First day of cycle: _____ . _____ . 20 _____   Thermometer: _________________

Cycle-Day	1	2	3	4	5	6	7	8	9	10	11	12	13	14	15	16	17	18	19	20	21	22	23	24	25	26	27	28	29	30	31	32	33	34	35	36	37	38	39	40
Bleeding																																								
Sex/intercourse (X)																																								
Cervical mucus **m = moist** **s = sticky** **e = eggwhite**																																								
Ovulation (O)																																								

My waking temperature in the morning (also known as basal temperature)

	1	2	3	4	5	6	7	8	9	10	11	12	13	14	15	16	17	18	19	20	21	22	23	24	25	26	27	28	29	30	31	32	33	34	35	36	37	38	39	40
37,5																																								
37,4																																								
37,3																																								
37,2																																								
37,1																																								
37,0																																								
36,9																																								
36,8																																								
36,7																																								
36,6																																								
36,5																																								
36,4																																								
36,3																																								
36,2																																								
36,1																																								
Time of measuring																																								

Cycle-Day	1	2	3	4	5	6	7	8	9	10	11	12	13	14	15	16	17	18	19	20	21	22	23	24	25	26	27	28	29	30	31	32	33	34	35	36	37	38	39	40
Alcohol?																																								
Party, late bedtime?																																								
Ill? Fever?																																								
Breast-feeding? (exclusive/complementary)																																								
Other notes																																								

Avoiding pregnancy or wanting to achieve one? Some stats on fertility:

Earliest high temperature reading in this cycle on day:

Earliest high temperature reading in all previous cycles including this one:

Deduct 8 to determine the start of your potentially fertile days = the earliest potentially fertile day so far:

Tip: Also record your ovulation day as per your own estimation and gut feeling, as well as the day determined by waking temperature, in the ovulation column. Some women are very aware of their ovaries around the time of ovulation (pulling or stabbing sensation on the right or left, just below the umbilicus). Additionally, around the time of ovulation, your cervical mucus is slippery-stretchy, almost liquid, similar to eggwhite.

Sanitary protection used in this cycle:

Pain levels and/or pain medication used in this cycle:

My experiences with freebleeding in this cycle:

Wishing to avoid/achieve pregnancy in this cycle:

Anything else of importance in this cycle:

Cycle number:

Shortest cycle so far: ________ days

Longest cycle so far: ________ days

Where was temperature taken:
Rectum ☐
Vagina ☐
Mouth ☐
Ear ☐

First day of cycle: _____ . _____ . 20 ____   Thermometer: _________________

Cycle-Day	1	2	3	4	5	6	7	8	9	10	11	12	13	14	15	16	17	18	19	20	21	22	23	24	25	26	27	28	29	30	31	32	33	34	35	36	37	38	39	40
Bleeding																																								
Sex/intercourse (X)																																								
Cervical mucus m = moist s = sticky e = eggwhite																																								
Ovulation (O)																																								

My waking temperature in the morning (also known as basal temperature)

37,5
37,4
37,3
37,2
37,1
37,0
36,9
36,8
36,7
36,6
36,5
36,4
36,3
36,2
36,1

Time of measuring

Cycle-Day	1	2	3	4	5	6	7	8	9	10	11	12	13	14	15	16	17	18	19	20	21	22	23	24	25	26	27	28	29	30	31	32	33	34	35	36	37	38	39	40
Alcohol?																																								
Party, late bedtime?																																								
Ill? Fever?																																								
Breast-feeding? (exclusive/ complementary)																																								
Other notes																																								

Avoiding pregnancy or wanting to achieve one? Some stats on fertility:

Earliest high temperature reading in this cycle on day:

Earliest high temperature reading in all previous cycles including this one:

Deduct 8 to determine the start of your potentially fertile days = the earliest potentially fertile day so far:

Tip: Also record your ovulation day as per your own estimation and gut feeling, as well as the day determined by waking temperature, in the ovulation column. Some women are very aware of their ovaries around the time of ovulation (pulling or stabbing sensation on the right or left, just below the umbilicus). Additionally, around the time of ovulation, your cervical mucus is slippery-stretchy, almost liquid, similar to eggwhite.

Sanitary protection used in this cycle:

Pain levels and/or pain medication used in this cycle:

My experiences with freebleeding in this cycle:

Wishing to avoid/achieve pregnancy in this cycle:

Anything else of importance in this cycle:

Cycle number: [ ]

Shortest cycle so far: _________ days

Longest cycle so far: _________ days

First day of cycle: _____ . _____ . 20 _____   Thermometer: _________________

Cycle-Day	1	2	3	4	5	6	7	8	9	10	11	12	13	14	15	16	17	18	19	20	21	22	23	24	25	26	27	28	29	30	31	32	33	34	35	36	37	38	39	40
Bleeding																																								
Sex/intercourse (X)																																								
Cervical mucus m = moist s = sticky e = eggwhite																																								
Ovulation (O)																																								

My waking temperature in the morning (also known as basal temperature)

37,5
37,4
37,3
37,2
37,1
37,0
36,9
36,8
36,7
36,6
36,5
36,4
36,3
36,2
36,1

Time of measuring

Cycle-Day	1	2	3	4	5	6	7	8	9	10	11	12	13	14	15	16	17	18	19	20	21	22	23	24	25	26	27	28	29	30	31	32	33	34	35	36	37	38	39	40
Alcohol?																																								
Party, late bedtime?																																								
Ill? Fever?																																								
Breast-feeding? (exclusive/complementary)																																								
Other notes																																								

Avoiding pregnancy or wanting to achieve one? Some stats on fertility:

Earliest high temperature reading in this cycle on day:

Earliest high temperature reading in all previous cycles including this one:

Deduct 8 to determine the start of your potentially fertile days = the earliest potentially fertile day so far:

Tip: Also record your ovulation day as per your own estimation and gut feeling, as well as the day determined by waking temperature, in the ovulation column. Some women are very aware of their ovaries around the time of ovulation (pulling or stabbing sensation on the right or left, just below the umbilicus). Additionally, around the time of ovulation, your cervical mucus is slippery-stretchy, almost liquid, similar to eggwhite.

Sanitary protection used in this cycle:

Pain levels and/or pain medication used in this cycle:

My experiences with freebleeding in this cycle:

Wishing to avoid/achieve pregnancy in this cycle:

Anything else of importance in this cycle:

Cycle number:

Shortest cycle so far: ________ days

Longest cycle so far: ________ days

Where was temperature taken:
Rectum ☐
Vagina ☐
Mouth ☐
Ear ☐

First day of cycle: _____ . _____ . 20 ____ Thermometer: ________________

Cycle-Day	1	2	3	4	5	6	7	8	9	10	11	12	13	14	15	16	17	18	19	20	21	22	23	24	25	26	27	28	29	30	31	32	33	34	35	36	37	38	39	40
Bleeding																																								
Sex/intercourse (X)																																								
Cervical mucus m = moist s = sticky e = eggwhite																																								
Ovulation (O)																																								

My waking temperature in the morning (also known as basal temperature)

| | 37,5 | 37,4 | 37,3 | 37,2 | 37,1 | **37,0** | 36,9 | 36,8 | 36,7 | 36,6 | 36,5 | 36,4 | 36,3 | 36,2 | 36,1 |

Time of measuring

Cycle-Day	1	2	3	4	5	6	7	8	9	10	11	12	13	14	15	16	17	18	19	20	21	22	23	24	25	26	27	28	29	30	31	32	33	34	35	36	37	38	39	40
Alcohol?																																								
Party, late bedtime?																																								
Ill? Fever?																																								
Breastfeeding? (exclusive/ complementary)																																								
Other notes																																								

Avoiding pregnancy or wanting to achieve one? Some stats on fertility:

Earliest high temperature reading in this cycle on day:

Earliest high temperature reading in all previous cycles including this one:

Deduct 8 to determine the start of your potentially fertile days = the earliest potentially fertile day so far:

Tip: Also record your ovulation day as per your own estimation and gut feeling, as well as the day determined by waking temperature, in the ovulation column. Some women are very aware of their ovaries around the time of ovulation (pulling or stabbing sensation on the right or left, just below the umbilicus). Additionally, around the time of ovulation, your cervical mucus is slippery-stretchy, almost liquid, similar to eggwhite.

Sanitary protection used in this cycle:

Pain levels and/or pain medication used in this cycle:

My experiences with freebleeding in this cycle:

Wishing to avoid/achieve pregnancy in this cycle:

Anything else of importance in this cycle:

Cycle number: [ ]

Shortest cycle so far: _________ days

Longest cycle so far: _________ days

Where was temperature taken:
Rectum ☐
Vagina ☐
Mouth ☐
Ear ☐

First day of cycle: _____ . _____ . 20 _____   Thermometer: _______________

Cycle-Day	1	2	3	4	5	6	7	8	9	10	11	12	13	14	15	16	17	18	19	20	21	22	23	24	25	26	27	28	29	30	31	32	33	34	35	36	37	38	39	40
Bleeding																																								
Sex/inter-course (X)																																								
Cervical mucus **m = moist** **s = sticky** **e = eggwhite**																																								
Ovulation (O)																																								

My waking temperature in the morning (also known as basal temperature)

		37,5
		37,4
		37,3
		37,2
		37,1
		37,0
		36,9
		36,8
		36,7
		36,6
		36,5
		36,4
		36,3
		36,2
		36,1

Time of measuring

Cycle-Day	1	2	3	4	5	6	7	8	9	10	11	12	13	14	15	16	17	18	19	20	21	22	23	24	25	26	27	28	29	30	31	32	33	34	35	36	37	38	39	40
Alcohol?																																								
Party, late bedtime?																																								
Ill? Fever?																																								
Breast-feeding? (exclusive/ complemen-tary)																																								
Other notes																																								

Avoiding pregnancy or wanting to achieve one? Some stats on fertility:

Earliest high temperature reading in this cycle on day:

Earliest high temperature reading in all previous cycles including this one:

Deduct 8 to determine the start of your potentially fertile days = the earliest potentially fertile day so far:

Tip: Also record your ovulation day as per your own estimation and gut feeling, as well as the day determined by waking temperature, in the ovulation column. Some women are very aware of their ovaries around the time of ovulation (pulling or stabbing sensation on the right or left, just below the umbilicus). Additionally, around the time of ovulation, your cervical mucus is slippery-stretchy, almost liquid, similar to eggwhite.

Sanitary protection used in this cycle:

Pain levels and/or pain medication used in this cycle:

My experiences with freebleeding in this cycle:

Wishing to avoid/achieve pregnancy in this cycle:

Anything else of importance in this cycle:

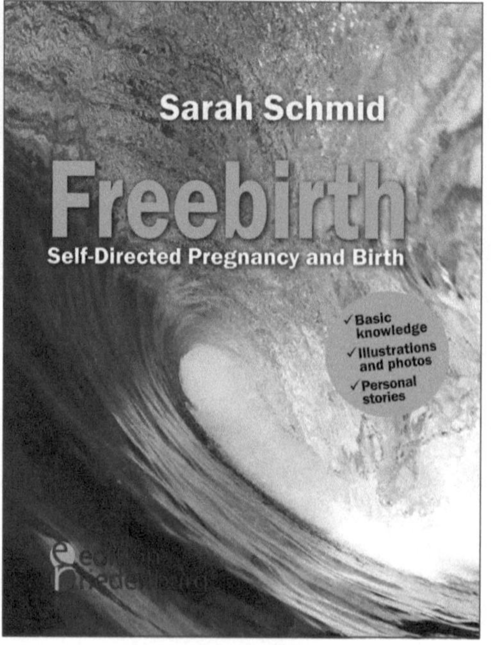

In 'Freebirth' Sarah Schmid – medical doctor and mother of five children – imparts a healthy amount of basic medical knowledge and dispels scary myths regarding birth. This also makes 'Freebirth' valuable for those women planning to birth their baby in a conventional setting as well as birth professionals.

Also in this book: Numerous illustrations • personal stories about planned and unplanned freebirths from 30 mothers including photos • helpful tips for the early days with your newborn

••• freebirth.me •••

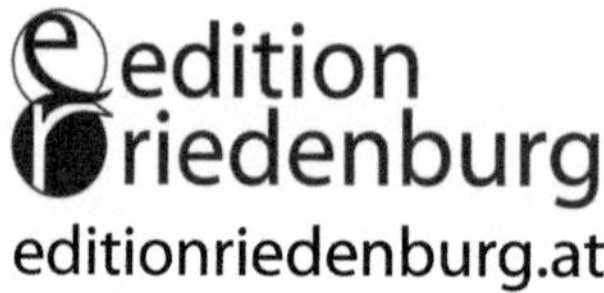

editionriedenburg.at